OPPORTUNITIES IN PUBLIC HEALTH CAREERS

George Pickett, M.D.
Terry W. Pickett

Foreword by
Iris R. Shannon, Ph.D., R.N.
President-Elect
American Public Health Association

VGM Career Horizons
A Division of National Textbook Company
4255 West Touhy Avenue
Lincolnwood, Illinois 60646-1975 U.S.A.

Cover Photo Credits:
Front cover: upper left and upper right,
National Institutes of Health; lower left and
lower right, *UCLA Public Health* Magazine.
Back cover: upper left, Centers for Disease
Control; upper right and lower left, National
Institutes of Health; lower right, UCLA School
of Public Health photo.

ABOUT THE AUTHORS

George Pickett, M.D., M.P.H., is a professor in the Department of Public Health Policy and Administration in the School of Public Health at the University of Michigan. Prior to that, he was chair of the Department of Health Care Organization and Policy in the School of Public Health at the University of Alabama at Birmingham.

Before entering the academic world of public health, Dr. Pickett was state health director of West Virginia. His other positions have included Director of Health and Welfare in San Mateo County, California, and Director of the Detroit/Wayne County Health Department. He holds a B.A. in government from Harvard University and received his medical degree at McGill University in Montreal, Canada. Dr. Pickett, with Dr. John Hanlon, is the coauthor of *Public Health: Administration and Practice,* a textbook widely used in schools of public health. He is past president of the American Public Health Association and the American College of Preventive Medicine and remains active in both organizations, as well as in many other public health organizations.

Terry Pickett, M.A., is currently a freelance writer in Ann Arbor, Michigan. Previously, she was a senior writer in the Office of University Relations at the University of Alabama at Birmingham.

Ms. Pickett holds a B.A. in history from Oberlin College and a master's degree in special education from the West Virginia

College of Graduate Studies. She has worked in the West Virginia Department of Health, where she wrote, edited, and produced *Health Trends,* the department's newsletter. She has also taught special education and worked as a houseparent at a residential school for developmentally disabled children near Edinburgh, Scotland.

ACKNOWLEDGMENTS

We would like to thank the following health departments for providing us with material about jobs in public health, without which this book could not have been written: Michigan Department of Health, Mississippi State Department of Health, Missouri Department of Health, New Mexico Health and Environment Department, Oklahoma State Department of Health, Rhode Island Department of Health, Virginia Department of Health, West Virginia Department of Health, Wisconsin Department of Health and Social Services, Akron (Ohio) City Health Department, Cincinnati (Ohio) Health Department, Genesee County (Michigan) Health Department, Jefferson County (Alabama) Department of Health, Kansas City (Missouri) Health Department, Kent County (Michigan) Health Department, Monterey County (California) Department of Health, Richmond (Virginia) City Health Department, Santa Barbara (California) Health Care Services, and Washtenaw County (Michigan) Health Department.

FOREWORD

As we enter the twenty-first century, the challenges and opportunities in public health are both exciting and limitless. Persons interested in discovery and in facilitating change should consider public health as a career option. In public health, opportunities for discovery and change are vested in goals directed toward reducing the risk of disease, disability, and premature death and toward improving the quality of life for all citizens. Public health workers value working with populations not only to achieve these goals but also to support them in becoming self-sufficient. The constant emergence of new or recurring national and international issues in public health creates an ongoing need for prepared and effective workers.

Approaches to the control and prevention of complex population problems such as teen suicide, AIDS, tuberculosis, teen pregnancy, sexually transmitted diseases, industrial accidents, or violence require solutions grounded in the public health sciences. Hence, preparation and practice in sciences which have a population focus such as epidemiology, biostatistics, public health administration, and other sciences distinguish the preparation of public health workers from other types of health workers. However, skills must also be developed in the ability to identify, assess, plan, and monitor an array of problems such as those related to access, availability, and utilization of health care; social and health policy issues; research and development; advocacy; and evaluation. Public health needs careerists committed to working with populations, particularly those populations at most risk of poor health.

To provide the context for exploration of public health as a career, the authors, George and Terry Pickett, have traced the beginnings of public health to its present organization and practice. They have clearly established government's responsibility for the public's health but have also established the public/private partnerships created to achieve public health objectives. Although emphasis was given to public health's focus on prevention of disease and the promotion of health, the reader is exposed to the broader implications of how these activities are carried out at the local, state, and federal levels. *Opportunities in Public Health Careers* is a stimulating effort which identifies a variety of multidisciplinary workers needed to achieve broad and complex public health goals. Hopefully, the readers will be motivated to further explore the varied and expansive opportunities in public health for a rewarding and challenging career.

Iris R. Shannon, Ph.D., R.N.
President-Elect
American Public Health Association

CONTENTS

organizations. The current status of federal public
health efforts.

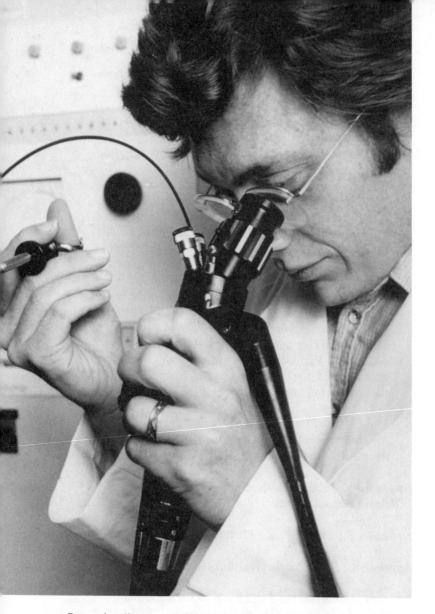

Preventing disease, prolonging life, and promoting health and efficiency through community effort are the goals of public health workers. (United States Department of Health and Human Services photo)

CHAPTER 1

WHAT IS PUBLIC HEALTH?

We live in a very safe world. In the United States, in spite of AIDS and cancer and heart disease, most of us can expect to live to the age of seventy-five or beyond. Things are not perfect; too many babies, especially those born to mothers who are poor, die during their first year of life, and too many teen-agers and young adults die due to gunshot wounds and other violence. In some countries people are faced with the threats of a badly polluted environment, a host of uncontrolled infectious diseases, and, at the same time, the modern plagues of heart disease, cancer, and alcoholism. Nonetheless, for those fortunate enough to live in a well-developed country, there are not many serious threats to health. We live in a sanitary world with many aspects of our lives carefully protected by laws and regulations.

It was not always so.

As recently as 1842, in England, Edwin Chadwick found that more than half of all children of the working class died before their fifth birthday. The average age at death was 36 for the gentry, 22 for tradesmen, and 16 for laborers.

How did this dramatic change in our health status and longevity occur? In large part it was due to the discoveries and practices of public health.

What is public health then? An early definition in a 1920 *Modern Medicine* article by C.-E. A. Winslow states that it is:

... the science and art of 1) preventing disease, 2) prolonging life, and 3) promoting health and efficiency through organized community effort for—

a. the sanitation of the environment,
b. the control of communicable diseases,
c. the education of the individual in personal hygiene,
d. the organization of medical and nursing services for the early diagnosis and preventive treatment of disease, and
e. the development of the social machinery to insure everyone a standard of living adequate for the maintenance of health, so organizing these benefits as to enable every citizen to realize his birthright of health and longevity.

A shorter definition of public health is that it involves the organization of public resources to prevent the dependency that would otherwise result from disease or injury.

THE ORIGINS OF PUBLIC HEALTH

The roots of public health are very old. Some of the dietary laws of the ancient Jews, as described in the Old Testament, were probably developed to prevent certain common diseases, even though the concept of microorganisms, such as bacteria and viruses, was not understood at all. Excavations at the sites of very primitive tribes show that they understood the need to draw their fresh water upstream from their campsite and to discard their wastes into the river downstream.

The Roman Empire

Different societies at different times in history felt that the state (society and its formal structure of governance) had no business regulating personal affairs. At other times, people supported extensive systems of regulation and control. During the height of the Roman Empire, the government was intimately involved in public health work, including the construction of sewers and a public water supply system, as well as making regulations concerning the sale of food, elimination of dangerous building conditions, the control of prostitution, and licensure of bakers.

The Dark Ages

After the Fall of Rome there was a general revulsion against the physicality of life. The luxuries of Rome were equated with sin. It was the spiritual side of life that counted. Throughout the long period of the Dark Ages, cleanliness was not considered next to godliness, but, rather, to Satan. Regulation of the environment was no longer thought to be important. Sewage and garbage were allowed to accumulate in the streets. Chamber pots were emptied out the windows when they were full, and sewage ran down an open ditch in the middle of the street. Foodstuffs were no longer controlled. Refrigeration was unknown. Many spices were used just to mask the smell of aging meat. The water supply was fouled with typhoid, cholera, and other noxious creatures. There was little, if any, effort made to prevent disease. Leprosy followed the routes of the Crusaders. Cholera followed the pilgrims to and from Mecca. The plague swept down out of China on the backs of the Mongols to invade the rest of the world.

The Black Plague

The plague was awesome. Caused by *Yersinia pestis,* a bacterium that infects the fleas on rats, it swept over Europe in waves from 1340 until the late 1700s, killing more than 60 million people. Called the Black Death, in the year 1348 it killed 60,000 people in Florence, 100,000 in Venice, 50,000 in Paris, and, in Vienna, 1,200 daily. As late as 1790, Marseilles and Toulon in France lost 70,000 people due to the plague in a time when cities were small compared to today's megalopolises. In Avignon, the churchyard was full; the Pope blessed the Rhone River so bodies could be thrown into it.

People attributed disease to personal vices, an act of God or the Devil, or to "vapors" or "humors" (gases and liquids in the environment and the body). Malaria (mal or "bad" air) was so named because it was believed that people who lived near stagnant, smelly water were likely to get the disease. The role of the mosquito and its microscopic parasite was not yet understood.

Yet some people seemed to have a crude understanding of contagion. In 1348 Venice banned entry of plague-infected ships, and, in 1383, Marseilles passed the first quarantine law. Under quarantine, people attempting to enter the community were held in a quarantine station until they were thought to be safe. No such attention was paid to the rat or its fleas, however.

The Renaissance

In the 1600s, according to one observer, ". . . one could wander ten miles without seeing a soul. . . . In every village, there are houses filled with dead bodies and carrion; men, women, children, servants, horses . . . lying pell mell together, throttled by plague and hunger. . . ."

As the plague receded, life changed, what was left of it. Artisans left their villages to join merchants in manufacturing such things as gloves and hats and guns. People began to gather together in cities to run the new machines of industry. The luxuries of Rome were no longer avoided; most people simply could not afford them, and others were too busy to enjoy them.

In the increasingly crowded towns and cities of Western Europe disease ran rampant in a filthy environment inhabited by people poorly fed, badly housed, and wretchedly clothed. The conditions of work were abominable, especially for children who were thought of as consumable resources. Look into a London workhouse in 1708 as described by M. D. George in *London Life in the Eighteenth Century:*

> . . . thirty or forty children were put under the charge of one nurse in a ward, they lay two together in bunks arranged round the walls in two tiers, "boarded and set one above the other . . . a flock bed, a pair of sheets, two blankets and a rug to each." Prayers and breakfast were from 6:30 to 7. At 7 the children were set to work, twenty under a mistress, "to spin wool and flax, knit stockings, to make new their linen,

clothes, shoes, . . . etc." This work went on till 6 PM with an interval from 12 to 1 for "dinner and play." Twenty children were called at a time for an hour a day to be taught reading, some also writing. Some children, we are told, "earn a halfpenny, and some fourpence a day." At twelve, thirteen or fourteen, they were apprenticed, being given, at the master's choice, either a "good ordinary suit of clothes or 20 shillings in money."

The Enlightenment

Slowly, as trade expanded and the early phases of the Industrial Revolution emerged, interest in the prevention of disease was reawakened. It was not charity or beneficence that made the difference. People were seen as a valuable resource of the state. They were useful both in wars and in manufacturing. It was important for the state to protect such a valuable resource.

The philosophical underpinnings of society were changing, too. It was the Age of Enlightenment. John Locke, Rousseau, John Stuart Mill, and others described a new, more egalitarian world in which people, all people, had a right to life, liberty, and the pursuit of happiness simply by virtue of the fact that they were human beings. It served the state well to improve the health of its citizens, but it served the spirit well, too.

New sanitary laws were passed governing the production and sale of food, housing, water supplies, air pollution, and even working hours and conditions. Concepts of quarantine were rediscovered and applied, even though no one yet understood what a bacterium or a virus was.

Then that changed too.

Nineteenth Century Discoveries

In the mid-1800s a succession of amazing discoveries changed forever the state's potential to intervene in the public's health. In 1850, John Snow of London deduced how cholera infected an entire community by examining the spread of the disease among different population groups using different water supply systems. This was the first scientific example of epidemiology, or the study of the distribution of disease in a population group—its origins, characteristics, and spread.

Epidemiology is the basic science and practice of public health. Virologists identified the virus of AIDS, but the epidemiologists were the ones who found the epidemic, identified the most likely victims, deduced its method of spread, and guided public efforts to control it. Epidemiologists first discovered the horrifying link of cigarettes to cancer. They studied groups of people (smokers and nonsmokers) rather than single patients.

Not long after that Pasteur discovered the concepts which made it possible to immunize people against some of the most common, serious diseases. Lister discovered antisepsis, which made the treatment of wounds possible and allowed surgery to be performed without causing death due to infection. It was an astonishing period, one which Osler said had ". . . made the century forever memorable."

The scientific tools were now available. The philosophy of the state began to change toward more democratic forms of government, and the people began to insist that their governments protect them from disease and injury.

PUBLIC HEALTH TODAY

With the convergence of science, philosophy, and societal consent, public health programs were established throughout Europe, the Mideast, the Far East, and in Africa for a variety of reasons: charity, selfishness, and concerns for equity. In most of the world, public health included programs intended to protect health and to prevent disease as well as to provide basic medical care services to those who were unable to pay for them. (The United States has a somewhat different emphasis which will be discussed in the next chapter.)

Today public health agencies provide services in almost every community of the world. They immunize us to prevent once common and deadly infectious diseases, keep records of when we're

born and when we die, and monitor our health if we should contract communicable diseases such as tuberculosis, syphillis, or
AIDS. They educate us to live more healthfully through nutrition,
stop-smoking, and exercise programs, and through disease prevention programs covering everything from arthritis and accident
prevention to breast self-examination and the early detection and
treatment of high blood pressure. They guard our food supplies,
protect our water, and keep environmental hazards under surveillance. They also provide needed medical services for many
people.

PUBLIC HEALTH AND MEDICAL CARE

The term *public health* implies that there is such a thing as private health. The true distinction, at least in the United States, is
between public health and medical care. Medical care seeks to
treat problems that have occurred—to cure disease. Public health
seeks to prevent the problems from occurring. In the United
States, medical care is basically a private matter, whereas public
health priorities and programs are determined in the public arena
to serve social or community needs. In many parts of the world
such distinctions are not understood, neither in theory nor in
practice, but the United States has had a unique history.

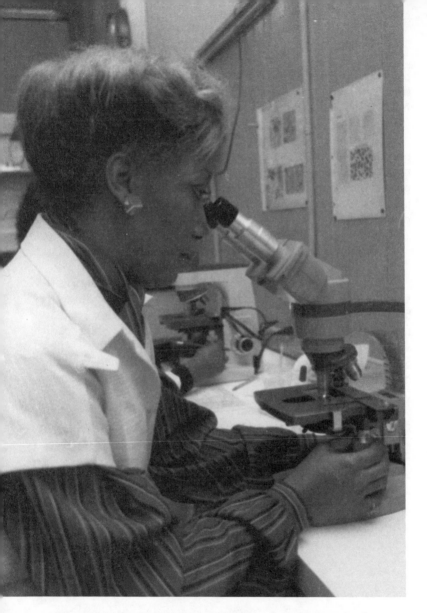

Researching diseases to prevent epidemics and provide cures has been a concern of public health practitioners throughout the history of the United States. (Chicago Department of Health photo)

CHAPTER 2

PUBLIC HEALTH IN THE UNITED STATES

Public health developed more slowly in the United States and took on a different shape than in Europe. By the mid-nineteenth century, public health in England and on the Continent encompassed not only protection and sanitation of the environment, but some medical care services for the populace as well. In American society, however, the *prevention* of disease and the *treatment* of disease were sharply separated. Two main factors appear to account for the divergent development of public health on each side of the Atlantic: different traditions of care-giving and the more rapid progress of medical science in Europe than in the United States. Public health, public medical care programs, and publicly supported mental health systems are separate entities in the United States.

PUBLIC MEDICAL CARE IN THE UNITED STATES

The first settlers in the New World were Protestants. They protested. They protested the intrusion of government into the privacy of their lives, their schools, their homes, and their businesses. The Catholic church had a strong tradition of caring, and most so-called hospitals in the 1600s in Europe were Catholic charitable institutions for the needy, aged, or infirm. There was little that could be done to treat disease, but caring was a religious act.

The Protestants were not Catholics; they did not bring such traditions with them. Charity began at home. It was not only *not* a sin to look after one's creature comforts, it was an obligation. The family came first—feeding it, clothing it, housing it, and protecting it. That required hard work and the accumulation of wealth.

Early Colonists

The early settlers carved out a new way of life. There was little need to waste precious resources on people who neither could nor would help themselves. No hospitals were established in colonial America. They were built in French Montreal to the north and Spanish Mexico City to the south since these were settled by Catholic countries, but not in what was to become the United States. Survival depended partly on the will of God and partly on one's own perseverance.

Medical care was not on the societal agenda for the early colonists, with the exception of efforts to prevent a sick person from infecting others. One's personal health was a private matter. It had little to do with the rest of the community and the rest of the community could do little to improve it.

Medical Education in Europe and America

It wouldn't have done the colonists much good to use medical care even if they had wanted to, for medical care in the colonies was abysmally bad. In some of the great European cities, the early signs of science and scholarship were becoming evident in the great medical schools, but there were no such schools on this side of the Atlantic, and very few trained physicians. The great biological discoveries that were revolutionizing medical education in Europe were slow to cross the Atlantic. In the United States the few existing professional teaching facilities were inadequate; many so-called physicians were self-proclaimed and itinerant. "Medicines" included remedies from medieval Europe, borrowings from native Americans, and homemade concoctions. They were generally so bad that one observer remarked, "If the whole materia medica as now used, could be sunk to the bottom of the sea, it would be all the better for mankind—and all the worse for the fishes."

Public Support in Europe and America

Little faith was placed in physicians. In the limited instances in which it was thought that a physician's care was needed, his or her services were cheap. In the 1870s, Dr. Hiram Buhrman practiced in small towns in Maryland and Pennsylvania. His usual fee was twenty-five cents for an office visit. He made home calls for fifty cents, delivered babies for five dollars, and extracted teeth for twenty-five cents apiece, unless several were pulled at the same time, in which case there was a discount. He used few instruments and compounded his own drugs. He did not use a hospital.

Unlike education, medical care had no public support. Why should society pay for something of so little demonstrable value? Health departments stuck to their concerns with the environment and prevention of disease. Medical practitioners were considered to be private entrepreneurs, like other business people, but not nearly as useful.

In Europe the situation was quite different. Science had progressed more rapidly; basic medical care services were often considered an appropriate activity for public health agencies. So much importance was attached to medical care that several European politicians supported some form of national health insurance in order to remain in power. By 1886, the German Chancellor Otto Von Bismarck had secured compulsory health insurance in Germany, and the pattern spread.

Improvements in America

The turn of the century saw the beginnings of remarkable improvements in American medical education. The superiority of the great European medical schools had become apparent. In 1904, the American Medical Association passed a resolution urging that young men obtain a high school diploma before entering medical school. In 1910, Sir William Osler and John Halstead, at Johns Hopkins University, were successful in introducing the new concept of a full-time salaried faculty with a four-year, after-college education in general medicine, followed by training in a specialized area such as surgery, medicine, or pediatrics.

Medical care in the United States soon came of age. American medical science and education made great advances with the advent of postgraduate medical education. That, coupled with the introduction of private health insurance two decades later, led to the development of the strongest, best-equipped, and wealthiest medical care system in the world.

By the 1930s, the American public believed that medical care was important. And by the end of the Second World War, they realized that medical care was no longer affordable for everyone. Since the 1950s, then, because of its value and cost, medical care has been a public policy issue.

Today, although American medicine has made possible the miracles of heart transplants, computers for eyes, and genetic engineering, too many people are receiving inadequate medical care. The United States has one of the highest infant mortality rates in the developed world. (The infant mortality rate is the number of deaths occurring in infants under one year of age per 1,000 live births. In the United States, it is currently about 11 per 1,000. In some countries it is as low as 9 per 1,000. In the black population of the United States, it is about 20 per 1,000.) Medical care costs continue to increase twice as fast as the costs of other goods and services. Medicare, which pays for much of the medical care used by people over the age of sixty-five, costs over $70.5 billion a year; Medicaid, a federal-state program to pay for necessary medical services for certain low income people, now spends more than $40 billion each year. A family can be wiped out financially by a major illness.

Many public medical care programs have been a function of the public welfare system, not public health. Only in the last twenty-five years has public health become aggressively involved in medical care, with public health agencies providing direct health care services through neighborhood or rural health centers in some instances, and lobbying for public health programs and regulation of health care costs on the political front. The relationship between medical care and public health, though closer than in the past, remains unclear.

PUBLIC MENTAL HEALTH IN THE UNITED STATES

In 1953, sociologist H. E. Jensen wrote, "If it isn't mental health, it isn't public health." Today most problems associated with mental illness—alcoholism, drug abuse, suicide, depression, and schizophrenia—are also considered public health problems. Yet because of their distinct histories, public health and mental health have established separate organizational structures and organizations with different goals and different methods of reaching those goals. Consequently, two fields that should be working harmoniously with each other are often at cross purposes.

Mental health, compared to public health and medicine, is a relatively new field. Not so long ago the mentally ill were hidden away in jails or asylums. Treatment was not thought worthwhile. The mentally ill were exhibited as freaks in sideshows, restrained in straight jackets or chains, beaten, or surgically pacified. Since no one knew what caused mental illness, preventive health services did not seem applicable; public health was not interested.

Large state-run hospitals were built for the incarceration of the mentally ill, supposedly for their own security and the community's. The hospitals were managed separately from the public health system, which was concerned with sanitation and the control of infectious diseases.

The Mental Health Movement

As was the case with medical care, mental health care was more advanced in Europe than in the United States. Agitation for more humane treatment of the mentally ill, to treat them as victims rather than criminals or witches, began at the end of the eighteenth century in France. Not until fifty years later did a similar movement emerge in the United States led by Dorothea Dix. The foundations of psychiatry and psychology were laid in the late nineteenth century, opening the way for preventive approaches to mental illness.

With the publication of Clifford W. Beers's book, *A Mind That Found Itself,* in 1908, the mental health movement began in earnest in the United States. Beers described graphically his experiences in several institutions for the mentally ill and concluded with a plea for drastic reform and education in mental health. Support was strong and immediate, enabling Beers to establish the Connecticut Society for Mental Hygiene, the first organization of its kind. In 1909, the National Committee for Mental Hygiene was organized. The first International Mental Hygiene Congress was held in Washington, D.C., in 1930.

In 1948, the National Institute of Mental Health, which was to become one of the premier mental health organizations in the world, was formed. Under its umbrella, hospital and research facilities have been built. It also provides consultation and aid to individual states to expand their own facilities and increase mental health personnel. Further legislation provided the funds to establish community mental health centers.

Modern Public Mental Health

After years of neglecting mental health, public health leaders finally began to realize its importance and relevance to their own field. But mental health, having gained acceptance and strength as a separate entity, insisted on maintaining that separation. Consequently, in most states and communities public mental health programs are organized and managed separately from the public health agencies. Often the responsibility for mental health programs is divided not only between public health and mental health, but among welfare, institutions, and special boards or commissions, too.

Effective mental health care for the community involves everyone from parents, family physicians, and the clergy, to psychologists, psychiatrists, public health nurses, psychiatric social workers and social scientists, epidemiologists, and statisticians. Coordination of the organizations is essential. Although progress has been made in the past twenty years, there is still much confusion in the delivery of mental health services to the consumer. The patient or client may get the counseling needed from the social worker, but not the medication needed from the public health nurse, or vice versa. Public health and mental health agencies must work even harder to develop more effective methods of coordination and cooperation.

PUBLIC HEALTH IN THE UNITED STATES

During the United States's infancy, most of its cities were on the seacoast. The citizens of those cities were concerned about the importation of plague, cholera, and smallpox. Occasionally a ship, passing in the night, would stealthily unload the pock-marked body of a sailor, living or dead, on the town's wharf to lessen the chance that the rest of the ship's crew would sicken and die. To protect themselves the town dwellers often built a pest house outside the town's limits in which to place the sick sailor until he died or recovered.

There were other worrisome problems. A horse would die in the city square or a bale of tea leaves would be left rotting on the wharf. These rotting bales and putrifying carcasses were believed to be the source of diseases. They were thought to give off vapors that could cause fevers. They had to be removed. A handyman was hired to haul off the dead carcass or the rotting bale and burn it or bury it outside of town—the forerunner of today's environmental health worker.

As early as 1647, the Massachusetts Bay Colony passed a regulation to prevent pollution of Boston Harbor. In 1701, Massachusetts passed laws for the isolation of smallpox patients and for ship quarantine. These and similar regulations passed in other colonies dealt with sanitation and attempted to prevent the spread of disease. But there was no ongoing group or organization to assure identification of problems in the first place, and no mechanism to enforce compliance with the regulations.

Not much progress was made in public health in colonial America throughout the rest of the century. The insightful Benjamin Rush, physician and American patriot, was far ahead of his time when he wrote that political institutions, economic organization, and disease were so interrelated that any general social change produced accompanying changes in health. Many people today still do not recognize this truism.

Early Boards of Health

After the American Revolution, and with the onslaught of one epidemic after another (Philadelphia had to be abandoned as the nation's capital because of a virulent yellow fever outbreak), interest became widespread in establishing local boards of health to advise the town fathers how to deal with the threat of pestilence. Boston, Philadelphia, Baltimore, and New York were among the first cities to establish local boards of health before the close of the eighteenth century. Their concerns, using the New York City public health committee as an example, included the "quality of the water supplies, construction of common sewers, drainage of marshes, interment of the dead, planting of trees and healthy vegetables, habitation of damp cellars, and the construction of a masonry wall along the water front."

Between 1800 and 1850, the United States grew by leaps and bounds, both in size and population. Public health, with its early efforts to control sanitation and the spread of disease, did not keep pace. Epidemics of smallpox, yellow fever, cholera, typhoid, and typhus occurred with frightening regularity. Tuberculosis and malaria were everyday facts of life. Twenty percent of the babies born in this period died before their first birthday. The average life expectancy in Boston and most older American cities was going down, not up.

The *Shattuck Report*

Into this morass of disease and ill health stepped Lemuel Shattuck, a layperson with an abiding interest in sanitary reform.

As a legislator in the Massachusetts state assembly, Shattuck constantly railed against the lack of progress in public health. He was appointed chairman of a legislative committee for the study of health and sanitary problems in the state. His previous occupations as teacher, historian, bookseller, sociologist, and statistician made him uniquely qualified for the task. The committee, with Shattuck as the primary author, produced in 1850 one of the most extraordinary documents in the history of public health: *Report of the Sanitary Commission of Massachusetts.* With its unpretentious title, the *Shattuck Report,* as it is called, laid the foundation for modern public health practice and organization. It was ahead of its time in 1850 (the report was virtually ignored until twenty-five years after its publication) and, sad to say, it is in many respects ahead of our time.

In the introductory statement of the report Shattuck proclaimed the committee's manifesto:

> We believe that the conditions of perfect health, either public or personal, are seldom or never attained, though attainable;—that the average length of human life may be very much extended, and its physical power greatly augmented;—that in every year, within this Commonwealth, thousands of lives are lost which might have been saved;—that tens of thousands of cases of sickness occur, which might have been prevented;—that a vast amount of unnecessarily impaired health, and physical debility exists among those not actually confined by sickness:—that these preventable evils require an enormous expenditure and loss of money, and impose upon the people unnumbered and immeasurable calamities, pecuniary, social, physical, mental and moral, which might be avoided;—that means exist, within our reach, for their mitigation or removal;—and that measures for prevention will effect infinitely more, than remedies for the cure of disease.

Shattuck opened his report with a review of public health progress in Europe, a record of major epidemics in Massachusetts, and statistics showing the decreasing life expectancy in Boston, Philadelphia, and New York.

Shattuck's Recommendations

With that as background Shattuck made fifty specific recommendations concerning the organization and mission of public health. Among them were the establishing of a state board of health and local boards of health in every city and town in the state (at a time when only a few local health departments with limited functions existed); the collection and analysis of vital statistics; developing a routine system for exchanging data and information; doing studies on tuberculosis; managing the control of alcoholism and supervision of mental disease; participating in town planning and building planning for a healthy environment; establishing nurses' training schools; training physicians in preventive as well as curative medicine; educating the public about public health programs and garnering its support; advising people to have routine physical examinations; and maintaining family records of illness.

Shattuck deduced the deleterious effects of air pollution on health. "Although we are as yet uninformed on this subject," he wrote, "it is unreasonable to suppose that we shall always remain so." The report also recommended that the contents of medicines be known and their effects observed, and that food adulteration be controlled, thus foreshadowing the primary responsibilities of today's Food and Drug Administration.

FORMATION OF LOCAL AND STATE HEALTH DEPARTMENTS

Although Lemuel Shattuck's report did not have an immediate effect, and progress in public health was slow, the number of local boards of health began to increase. Some boards began to hire staffs to carry out the functions assigned to the local boards, the first step in the formation of local health departments. Baltimore had one of the first, established in 1798. Other major cities followed suit throughout the nineteenth century. Their main functions were still reactive: to eliminate gross sanitary nuisances and prevent the spread of disease. The development of rural, or county, health departments came later, beginning in 1911.

Massachusetts was the first state to establish a state board of health in 1869, a direct, albeit delayed, response to the *Shattuck Report*. The concerns of the state health department were far broader than those at the local level. They included public and professional health education, housing conditions, studies of various diseases and measures for prevention, the sale of poisons, and conditions of the poor. The Massachusetts Health Department also began an exchange with local boards of health, trying to ascertain their powers and duties and collecting data for publication on the number and causes of deaths in the largest towns and cities. The state agency asked that each community designate a physician as correspondent. This correspondence is considered the basis of the cooperation between state and local health authorities that continues today.

By the end of the nineteenth century, forty states had full-time health departments. The remaining states established health departments in the early years of the twentieth century.

FEDERAL BEGINNINGS OF PUBLIC HEALTH

Public health at the national level developed separately from the local and state levels. Its initial task was very different, too. It, in fact, had to do with medical care, though it took a different course from private medical care.

The Marine Hospital Service

Early in its history the United States had a vigorous maritime trade. The new Congress was worried about merchant sailors who might become sick and have no family or other means of support in a port of call. To provide some means of caring for such individuals, one of the earliest acts of Congress in 1798 was to establish the Marine Hospital Service. Twenty cents a month was deducted from each sailor's pay to finance the services of physicians in port cities who were appointed to the service by the president. This was the first pre-paid medical and hospital insurance plan in the western world. Within two years the first marine hospital was built in Norfolk, Virginia, soon followed by others throughout the country.

As the nineteenth century progressed, the authority of the Marine Hospital Service expanded. States asked Marine Hospital Service physicians to help control local epidemics. The service was given the power of quarantine to prevent the onset or spread of epidemics. In 1890, Congress gave the Marine Hospital Service authority to inspect all immigrants for disease. Personnel of the service were given quasi-military status and provided with commissions and uniforms.

At about the same time, the Marine Hospital Service established its first research facility, a one-room laboratory of hygiene in the Marine Hospital on Staten Island in New York. In 1939, this small laboratory evolved into the National Institutes of Health, soon to become the largest and most prestigious medical research establishment in the world.

Congress, recognizing the greatly broadened responsibilities of the Marine Hospital Service, renamed it the Public Health and Marine Hospital Service in 1902. In 1912, it was renamed the United States Public Health Service, which is today the most important federal health agency.

The American Public Health Association

Shortly before the Civil War, health officers of major United States cities and others interested in public health attended a series of four meetings called the national Quarantine Conventions. Their purpose was to offer a forum to discuss matters of common concern related to disease prevention. Topics ranged from prevention of epidemic diseases such as cholera and yellow fever, to the importance of stagnant and putrid water, to filthy bedding. This initial effort to establish a national, more unified approach to public health was brought to a halt by the Civil War.

The desire for coordination and cooperation in public health matters was strong, however. After the Civil War those same public health leaders established the American Public Health Association in 1872, now the oldest and largest public health association in the world, with twenty-three sections representing health workers in maternal and child health, the environment, disease control, dental health, medical care, health administration, statistics, social work, nursing, mental health, and other important areas of interest.

PUBLIC HEALTH TODAY

The scope of public health in the United States has broadened enormously since the beginning of the twentieth century. Two world wars, a major economic depression, an increasingly complex society, and a better educated public have made public health more important than ever before.

From its watchdog protection/sanitation role, public health has grown to encompass areas as varied as prevention of both chronic and infectious diseases, indigent care, air pollution control, AIDS research, safety in the workplace, solid waste disposal, and much more.

With the Social Security Act of 1935 authorizing the United States Public Health Service to assist states in establishing and maintaining adequate public health services, and with the health legislation passed in 1965 during Lyndon Johnson's presidency, especially Medicare and Medicaid, the role of the federal government in public health grew rapidly. State and local health departments became dependent on federal funding. Federal, state, and local agencies each have their own structures and responsibilities, yet as they become more interdependent their functions seem to blend.

The American public health system is difficult to coordinate. The relationships of federal, state, and local agencies are in a state of change with leadership in health policy shifting from the federal government back to the states. Many local health departments have a broadly expanded mandate.

The separation of medical care, public health, mental health, and environmental health creates serious problems of continuity, effectiveness, and efficiency.

As the tasks become more complex and more important, better trained workers have become even more essential, and the role of the governmental presence in health has become increasingly important.

CHAPTER 3

THE GOVERNMENTAL PRESENCE IN HEALTH

In every community of the United States there is a governmental presence in health. It may not be especially vigorous or even effective in some places, but somewhere, in each community, there is an individual, usually appointed by a mayor, governor, or a board of health, whose job it is to see to it that the basic services of public health are available and in working order. Customarily, that individual has been called the "health officer" of the city, county, or state. There is not, however, a health officer for the nation.

The governmental presence in health is a concept used to describe those basic, preventive health services to which all people are entitled. Assuming there is some agreement about what those basic health services are (immunizations, for example, or protection of the water supply, food inspection, maternal and child health services), since they are considered to be rights, some agency of government must be responsible for assuring access to them. That is the difference between a privilege and a right; rights are guaranteed by the government.

It is not necessary that the person who represents the governmental presence in health have the direct responsibility for providing those services through the official public health department; they may be provided by a wide variety of public and private agencies, including the school system, the agriculture department, an environmental protection agency, the emergency medical services squad at one of the local hospitals, or a special district for sewage treatment and disposal. But there is in every community, or there should be, an individual trained in public health, whose job it is to be sure that such services are available, acceptable, and accessible.

BASIC PREVENTIVE HEALTH SERVICES

The basic services, those services that are thought to be of such value that they should be universally available, are not the same everywhere. Different states, and different communities within each state, have different lists. Some are quite extensive, some quite limited. They are not always written down in some convenient location either. State laws define certain activities, but many others have been developed to meet local needs in an innovative fashion. Some of the basic services of public health exist in what might be referred to as a form of common law. That is, their practice or availability has become assumed over time so that they are very much a part of the unwritten social compact that exists in every community.

It is not possible to list such services for every community because of the differences that exist. But one useful version of such a list is contained in a 1974 policy statement of the American Public Health Association. It includes the following:

Community Health Services
- Communicable disease control
- Chronic disease control (diabetes, heart disease, cancer)
- Rehabilitation services
- Family health services, including prenatal, well child, crippled children, school health, and family planning programs
- Dental health services (especially preventive health services such as water fluoridation, dental health education, and the use of sealants and fluoride mouthwashes in schools)
- Substance abuse services, including services for alcoholism and other drug abuse problems
- Accident prevention

- Nutrition services and education

Environmental Health Services
- Food protection
- Protection against hazardous substances such as chemicals and toxic wastes
- Protection of the drinking water supply
- Treatment and disposal of liquid wastes such as sewage
- Water pollution control
- Inspection and safety of recreational areas such as swimming pools, beaches, and parks
- Occupational health and safety
- Radiation protection
- Air quality control
- Noise pollution control
- Vector control (mosquitoes and stray animals, for example)
- Solid waste control
- Institutional sanitation (schools, prisons, and hospitals for the mentally ill)
- Housing sanitation and safety

Mental Health Services
- Prevention of mental disorders
- Consultation to community organizations such as schools and private social agencies
- Diagnostic and treatment services such as outpatient services, inpatient services, emergency services, day-care services, aftercare services, and diagnostic and evaluation services for the developmentally disabled

Personal Health Services
- Medical care services for special groups and those without the resources to obtain needed care for themselves and their families
- Health facilities operations such as county and city hospitals
- Emergency medical services
- Home health services
- Employee health programs
- Medical care for inmates of prisons and other institutions

Coordinating and Managing Functions
- Health data acquisition and processing
- Interagency planning
- Comprehensive state and regional health planning
- Disaster planning
- Health education of the public
- Health advocacy
- Continuing education of health personnel
- Research and development
- Organizing the health agency itself
- Policy analysis and direction
- Staffing the health agency
- Financial management of the health agency
- Liaison with other health agencies (federal, state, and local)

That is a long list. If you have read it carefully, you will find some things that you do not believe are done in your community, or you may find some things on the list that you know are the responsibility of some agency other than the health department. (You may also notice that the list provides a pretty good idea of the kinds of careers that can be found in public health.)

THE UNIQUENESS OF PUBLIC HEALTH

The list points out one other important characteristic of public health: its uniqueness. It is unlike any other organization in government. Almost all organizations, whether they are businesses, government agencies, or clubs, obtain their coherence, the stuff that glues them together, either from a common input process or skill or from a shared economic interest in the activity. A highway department centers around engineering and construction. The school board, while it hires drivers, cooks, and mechanics, as well as teachers, is devoted to the primary activity of education. The American Medical Association and the National League for Nursing stick together because their members have a common educational background and because they work in systems that have their own sort of economic rules and rewards.

Public health agencies, however, do not have a common, central discipline. Prevention of disease is a complex phenomenon that depends on a multitude of disciplines from law to nuclear physics, from medicine to engineering, from social work to statistics. The "glue" that holds public health together as an organization is its intended *outcome*: the prevention of disease and disability.

Virtually all agencies of the government have a role to play in public health: the police and fire departments, the schools, agriculture departments, economic development agencies, natural resources departments, libraries, highway departments, and the civil service system. That is what makes public health such a unique enterprise, and that is what makes it necessary to locate and understand the governmental presence in health. Public health agencies, no matter how large, cannot perform all of the activities of public health. They must depend upon the ability and the collaboration of numerous other agencies, most of whom have some other primary mission. It is the task of the governmental presence in health to ensure that the agreed upon standards are met. It was not always so complex a task.

THE BEGINNINGS OF HEALTH DEPARTMENTS

The first public health agencies in the United States developed in port cities such as Philadelphia, Boston, and Charleston, South Carolina. That was where most of the people lived, and that was where most of the epidemics began. Only later, much later, did the states begin to develop public health agencies.

Originally, the states were more representative of the people in rural areas than those who lived in cities. The cities had their own traditions and governments. But as more immigrants and new industry turned villages into small towns, the problems of modern urban life became more apparent and the benefits of public health services were better known by then. The *Shattuck Report* described the problems in vivid detail, and suggested the sorts of solutions that the states could and should consider. The notion of state intervention was still so new that it lay dormant for another twenty-five years. But beginning in the 1870s, one state after another established a public health department to prevent communicable diseases, to place the hazards of life under continuing surveillance, and to protect people from their environment.

GOVERNMENTS' ROLES IN PUBLIC HEALTH

The State's Role

The states were, and are, supreme in public health matters. In a federal system of government, there is an agreement, the Constitution, specifying the functions of the federal government and its principal subdivisions, the states. In our case, the body of the Constitution spells out the workings and powers of the federal government, including the responsibility to collect taxes to promote the common welfare and to regulate commerce between the states. These are the only provisions in the United States Constitution that empower the federal government to intervene in public health matters. The Tenth Amendment to the Constitution, the last of the rights in the Bill of Rights, states that all powers and functions of government that are not assigned to the federal government are reserved for the states. Those powers and functions include the police power functions of government (to prevent polluters from polluting, restaurants from serving contaminated food, and people with diseases from infecting other people) and the welfare functions (the provision of medical care to those who are too poor to be able to afford it for themselves and their families).

Generally speaking, federal workers are not able to enter a state and inspect restaurants or provide immunizations for children, inspect work sites, or set up medical care programs in urban or rural ghettos. They must depend on the states for such activities, although the federal government can (and does) collect taxes and offers to help pay for such services if the states wish to provide them. In this form of government—federalism—the states are supreme in public health matters.

Local governments, such as cities and counties, do not have the same relationship to their state governments as do the states to the federal government. The state-local relationship is not guided by principles of federalism. Cities do have charters or constitutions that enable them to perform most functions of government that are not prohibited by state law. Even so, those charters are granted by the state and can be revoked by the state. Counties, on the other hand, are administrative subdivisions of the state. They can do only what state law expressly allows them to do.

The County's Role

County governments developed later than city and state governments, and it has been only within the past two decades that they have taken on a larger and more sophisticated role in the United States. The first county health departments were established in 1911 (Guilford County, North Carolina, and Yakima County, Washington). The relationships of the local health departments to the state vary from state to state. Gradually, the city health departments have been folded into the county government structure in all except the largest cities. They were simply too expensive for smaller cities to maintain. Moreover, residents of the cities pay county property taxes, which are used to support the county health department, and city taxes to support the city health department as well. So it made sense, in many cities, to discontinue their health departments and rely upon county health departments for services. County health departments have become larger and more effective. Their role and their relationship to the state health agency vary a great deal from state to state, however.

In some states, such as Florida, Tennessee, and Mississippi, there are no "county public health departments," as that term is usually understood. There are, rather, county or district offices of the state public health agency. All public health workers are employees of the state, and all are accountable to the state health officer. The counties may or may not have any obligation to support those local branches of the state health agency. Often they choose to provide local tax revenues in order to have the services their citizens want and need.

In other states, such as California and New York, there is a long tradition of strong, well-managed local health departments. These are created pursuant to state laws, but they are governed by the county board of commissioners or a county board of health. They hire their own health officer and other employees and, within the limits and requirements of state law, pass their own ordinances and develop their own policies. These are states with relatively autonomous county health departments.

In many other states, the patterns are mixed. In Michigan, Nebraska, and Alabama, for example, the larger, more populated counties tend to have their own "autonomous" health departments, but the more rural counties are dependent on the state health department for their governmental presence in health. A career in local public health may involve working for a county, city, or state.

Autonomous Health Departments

Autonomy is a relative concept. As noted earlier, local governments are "inferior" to state governments in their independence. No local health department is truly autonomous. If a serious problem erupts, the state health agency can intervene. Nor is there a significant difference in the quality of the work performed in local health departments that are "autonomous" versus those that are a part of state government. Florida and Tennessee have outstanding, state-run local health units. New York and California have highly regarded and highly autonomous local health departments. In all four of those states, funding for local public health services is a shared state-local responsibility, even though their governance is different, and the basic services of the governmental presence in health are more or less the same.

STATE AND LOCAL HEALTH DEPARTMENTS IN THE 1980s

In 1985, the last year for which figures are available, state and local health departments spent more than $8.4 billion. Actually, no one knows how much was really spent. The figures published refer to the expenditures made by the state health agencies and those local health agencies about which the state knows something. Many local health departments do not report such information to the state. Moreover, a great deal of money is spent on public health activities outside of state and local public health agencies.

For example, in most states, the principal mental health agency is separate from the public health department. In forty-one states, the Medicaid program, which pays for some of the medical care needed by poor people, is operated by the welfare department, not public health. (In 1985, state Medicaid agencies spent more than $40 billion.) In many states, most of what once were considered to be environmental health programs are carried out by state environmental protection agencies or departments of natural resources. These expenditures are not reported by the state public health agencies.

Nonetheless, given that the estimates considerably understate the local health agency's effort in public health, they do provide a reasonable approximation of the programs of the state health agencies. Of the $8.4 billion, $5.4 billion was spent directly by the state health agencies on programs managed by them; $1.4 billion was made available to local health departments by the state agencies for local public health activities; and $1.6 billion was the amount raised and spent locally by those local health agencies that reported such information to their state agencies. (Again, that understates the amount spent by local health agencies since a lot of their work is not reported to their state agencies.)

STATE HEALTH AGENCIES

The state health agencies employ more than 120,000 people in a wide variety of categories. Some, such as epidemiologists and public health nurses, are unique to public health. Others, such as clerical personnel, practicing physicians, and accountants, are in job classifications common to many organizations.

Some state health agencies are free-standing agencies responsible directly to the governor or to a board of health (usually appointed by the governor), while others are part of a superagency, usually including social service functions and often including a wide variety of other state programs, such as mental health, probation, rehabilitation, and substance abuse.

Local Health Departments

In forty-five states and in Puerto Rico, there are 2,925 local health departments. (In the other five states, there are no local public health departments; the services are provided by the state directly.) Most of the population of the United States is covered by local health departments, but they vary enormously in size, from such very large agencies as the New York City Department of Health, to small, three-person (one nurse, one sanitarian, and one clerk) health departments operating out of the basements of county court houses in many rural areas.

PUBLIC HEALTH EXPENDITURES

The money to pay for public health services comes from state and local taxes, grants-in-aid from the federal government, revenues and fees for services, and grants from private foundations and other sources. In 1985, the amounts were as follows:

Total (in millions)	$8,405
State funds	3,774
Federal grants and contracts	2,638
Local funds	1,204
Fees	491
Other	297

Personal Health Services

The money was spent on a wide variety of services and activities. A little more than $5.7 billion dollars was spent on personal health services. Much of that (nearly $2.3 billion) was spent on maternal and child health services, including the giant WIC program, which provides needed food to low-income mothers and their young children, as well as pregnant women. (WIC is an acronym for the Supplemental Nutrition Program for Women, Infants and Children.) But significant amounts were spent on communicable disease control programs, dental health, programs to control chronic diseases such as high blood pressure, and mental health and substance abuse programs. Such activities employ a wide range of professional, technical, and administrative workers, including psychiatrists, pediatricians, nurses, epidemiologists, disease control investigators, dentists, nutritionists, social workers, and managers.

The number of people who receive such services, and the volume of service delivery, is astonishing. Nearly a third of the population receives one or more personal health services from various public health programs each year. This includes immunizations, prenatal care, pediatric and well child care, as well as screening for high blood pressure and cancer, and treatment of sexually transmitted diseases. Public health agencies, as a system, are the largest providers of health care services in the nation.

Health Resources Functions

The second largest expenditure effort ($627 million) was for what are called health resources functions. These include the development of needed health services, regulatory programs, such as hospital and nursing home licensure, vital and health statistics collection and analysis, and comprehensive health planning. These programs involve epidemiologists, statisticians, lawyers, planners, nurses, physicians, social workers, nutritionists, and environmentalists.

Environmental Health Programs

State and local health departments spent more than $658 million on environmental health programs in 1985, including functions such as consumer protection, general sanitation, water quality control, air pollution, waste management, occupational health and safety, and radiation control. Such activities require chemists, physicists, meteorologists, engineers, sanitarians, toxicologists, epidemiologists, statisticians, and industrial hygienists. Requirements for such specialists are increasing each year and other agencies have needs for environmental health workers as well.

Laboratory Programs

Laboratory programs are a big part of the work of state and local health agencies. They include general purpose laboratories for bacterial and viral examination, the production of vaccines (in two states), environmental labs involved in the identification of minute amounts of harmful chemicals, and, sometimes, the forensic laboratories that are involved in the investigation of crime.

General Functions

Finally, the state and local public health agencies spend a significant proportion of their funds (more than a half billion dollars in 1985) on the general functions of the governmental presence in health: maintaining surveillance of community health status, working with other agencies at the state and local levels to correct problems and improve programs, and educating the public about disease prevention and health promotion. These activities require public health administrators, planners, lawyers, nurses, physicians, educators, and policy analysts.

THE FUTURE OF HEALTH DEPARTMENT PROGRAMS

What will happen to these programs in the next ten to twenty years? Some health department programs have gotten smaller over the past two decades. Many environmental health functions have been moved into new and different agencies as circumstances have changed. We are less concerned now about the general sanitation of the environment and more involved in complex chemical and physical pollution management activities. The enormous problem of disposing of our wastes—hazardous wastes, garbage and liquid wastes, such as sewage—has finally become apparent in a society that uses more than 60,000 different chemicals daily.

The creation of new environmental protection agencies has caused some problems, and many states are figuring out ways to reinsert the skills and expertise of public health workers into the regulatory process. Environmental health work will clearly expand in the years ahead.

Health departments have also seen a reduction in the number of public health nurses employed as more people have become better able to care for their own health problems, and an increasing number of working people have acquired health insurance for themselves and their families. But the limits of that process are becoming more apparent. Most states are now wrestling with the problem of providing and paying for needed medical care services for people who are unable to purchase them—a growing proportion of people in this country. For many years the attempt has been made to buy health services for low income and other people with access problems in the open market—in private physicians' offices and hospitals. But it is becoming increasingly obvious that this "insurance" style approach cannot solve the entire problem. No matter how such systems are designed, some people end up with no protection at all, and many others have only partial protection. In many areas, local health departments have taken on a significant role in organizing and providing medical services for needy people. This role will expand in the future.

Public health work is becoming more and more complex. The problems are more complex, and so are the solutions. In keeping with its uniquely multidisciplinary approach to the prevention of disease and disability, public health work in the future will become even more complex and interactive as the governmental presence in health seeks to find new and better ways to orchestrate the resources of government to meet the public's needs and expectations.

Such work will continue to require not only skilled and sophisticated health workers, but also increasingly well-trained managers, planners, and leaders.

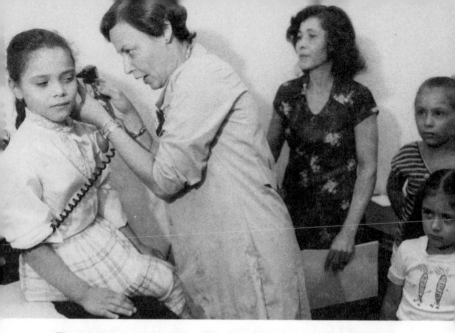

Top: A public health physician examines school children to ensure that they meet the legal requirements for examinations and immunizations. (Chicago Department of Health photo) *Bottom:* A sanitarian tests the water chemistry of a public swimming pool for compliance with public health codes. (County of Los Angeles Department of Health Services photo)

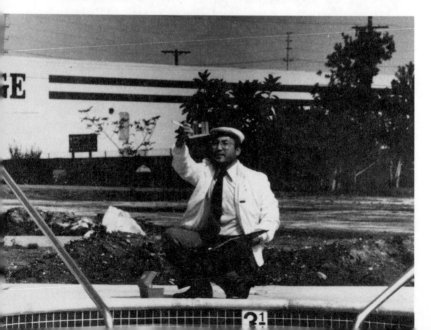

CHAPTER 4

PUBLIC HEALTH AT THE NATIONAL LEVEL

There is not a national health officer in the United States, nor is there a governmental presence in health. In this particular federal system of government, the responsibilities that would be involved in such a role or presence belong to the states. Nevertheless, the federal government has played a very important role in public health in the United States.

As at the state and local levels, there is one federal agency, the United States Department of Health and Human Services, which serves as the lead agency in health affairs. But there are numerous other agencies that have important roles to play: the Department of Education, the Department of Agriculture, the Department of Defense, the Environmental Protection Agency, the Department of Labor, the Veterans Affairs Administration, and even the State Department. Because of the federal nature of the United States government, the roles played by these national agencies are different from those carried out by their state and local counterparts.

THE CONSTITUTIONAL BASIS FOR A FEDERAL ROLE IN PUBLIC HEALTH

The word *health* does not appear in the United States Constitution. For reasons discussed in chapter 2, it was not considered to be an appropriate concern for the new federal government. Such matters, along with police protection and local schools, were left to the states. But the Constitution did contain some provisions which proved to be of considerable importance.

Promoting the General Welfare

The Preamble to the Constitution contains general language about the purpose of the document: "We the people of the United States, in order to form a more perfect union, establish justice, insure domestic tranquility, provide for the common defense, *promote the general welfare,* and secure the blessings of liberty to ourselves and to our posterity do ordain and establish this Constitution of the United States of America." While no specific provisions were made to carry out the intention, the language does indicate that at least one of the concerns of the federal government was the general welfare of the people. That phrase served to support presidential and congressional initiatives in Medicare, mental health, child health, alcoholism, and a host of other activities in the twentieth century.

Two other constitutional phrases have been of importance, both found in Article I, Section 8, where some of the powers of Congress were enumerated, including ". . . the power to lay and collect taxes [to] . . . provide for the common defense *and general welfare* of the United States . . ." and the power to ". . . regulate commerce . . . among the several states. . . ." The first of those two clauses has resulted in programs that are responsible for expenditures of more than $136 billion in 1986. The second clause, concerning the regulation of commerce between the states, has made possible the regulation of child labor, the control of drugs and vaccines, and the establishment of standards for workplace safety.

Regulating Interstate Commerce

The interstate commerce clause exemplifies the evolutionary nature of the federal role in public health. The framers of the Constitution did not intend for the federal government to become actively involved in the regulation of commerce between the states, but they were apprehensive about the possibility of trade wars between the states caused by the erection of barriers through the use of tariffs and other legal maneuvers. In order to prevent that from happening, the regulation of such matters was preempted, that is, taken from the states and assigned to the new federal government with the expectation that such powers would rarely, if ever, be exercised.

A century later, social welfare groups and labor unions pressed for federal legislation that would restrict the use of child labor. At first the Supreme Court ruled that the federal government lacked the power to interdict child labor. Gradually, over the years, attitudes changed, until finally the courts upheld the use of the interstate commerce clause to ban the use of child labor in any commercial enterprise that involved interstate commerce. In more recent years, such powers have been expanded considerably.

Collecting Taxes

The power to collect taxes in order to provide for the general welfare made possible the passage of the Medicare and Medicaid laws in 1965, which now pay for part of the medical care used by nearly one out of every four Americans, and expenditures of more than $120 billion in 1986.

Why the Government Was Slow to Become Involved

There are really two reasons, possibly three, the federal government was slow to become directly involved in the provision of health care services and in programs to prevent disease. First is the limited role of the federal government in matters involving the police power and welfare functions of government. While federal agencies have acquired some authority to become involved, their involvement has evolved gradually, and it is still generally assumed, by many people, that such matters are the province of the states.

Second, the federal government lacks a "delivery system" for public health. There is a governmental presence in health in every community of the United States, consisting of health officers, nurses, sanitarians, administrative personnel, and others. They work for state and local health departments, and are capable of contacting nearly every citizen, visiting every restaurant, inspecting every dairy plant, and working with every school at a moment's notice. They provide an enormous array of services.

The only similar service operated by the federal government has been the Postal Service. If the national government were to attempt to become involved in providing immunizations against communicable diseases directly, it would have to employ hundreds of thousands of workers, rent or build buildings, buy cars, computers, desks, and chairs, develop supervisory and administrative personnel, and get to know every community agency—a formidable task. It is far easier to try to work with the state and local health agencies to achieve federal objectives than to try to supplant them or compete with them.

Finally, partly because of the first and second reasons, but also for ideological reasons, many elected officials in the federal government would not want to open the door to such federal intervention. This has been especially apparent during the years of the Reagan administration.

GRANTS-IN-AID

Lacking the authority and/or the will to intervene more directly, Congress and the president have often sought to alter or stimulate state and local public health programs through the use of grants-in-aid. Grants-in-aid are offers of money from a larger to a smaller government to help the smaller government do something that both governments are interested in doing. For example, high blood pressure (known as hypertension) is a very common and serious health problem in the United States. It affects millions of people and often leads to complications, such as stroke (damage to the brain either by a broken blood vessel or one that is blocked with fatty deposits) and kidney disease. Some states became interested in the problem in the 1950s and, subsequently, the federal government came to the conclusion that a great deal could be done to control high blood pressure and its complications. Lacking the ability to become directly involved and recognizing the extensive network of trained workers available through state and local health departments, the United States Public Health Service offered grants of money to aid interested states in controlling high blood pressure.

With the money came certain conditions concerning its use: the need to focus on particular high risk groups, the use of a standardized method for measuring blood pressure, the collection of data in a uniform manner, and the reporting of that data to the federal granting agency. No state had to apply for and use such a grant, but if it did, it had to observe the conditions attached to the grant by the federal program managers. In most states, one or more agencies could be found with an interest in the program, and federal standards and guidelines thus became widely diffused throughout the country.

Benefits of Grants

Similar grants have been developed to deal with problems such as lead poisoning, sudden infant death syndrome, and rat control, as well as broad concerns such as mental health, maternal and child health, and medical care for the poor, which is covered by the Medicaid program. No state had to have a Medicaid program. However, all states have a constitutional responsibility (required by their own constitutions, not the federal Constitution) for the protection of those who cannot take care of themselves. Given the enormous expense of medical care, the availability of a federal grant meant a great deal. States were offered up to ninety percent of the cost of paying for such medical care if they developed and administered their programs in keeping with federal regulations. The percentage of the total cost paid by the federal government varied depending on the number of poor people in the state and the availability of state and local tax dollars to pay for the care. All states now have Medicaid programs, and all of the programs follow federal guidelines. Thus, while the federal program managers may have never entered a state nor seen a client, and while they were specifically prohibited from doing anything to alter the way in which medical care was practiced in the states, their influence has been enormous. (For more information, see *The Social Transformation of American Medicine* by Paul Starr, an excellent and very readable book.)

Grants-in-aid have been significant in the development of public health in the United States. By 1981, there were more than 200 federal grants-in-aid programs involving more than 150 different Washington bureaus. (Not all of these were health grants. Grants were made for education systems, highways, agriculture, and a host of other activities.) Altogether, health grants-in-aid to state and local health departments amounted to $2.6 billion in 1985. (The states spent $3.8 billion dollars of their own funds.)

Disadvantages of Grants

But such grants are not always welcomed. Their availability has often enticed communities to become involved in activities that would not otherwise have been considered high on their list of important things to do. They have also, at times, encouraged communities to invest in facilities and equipment that they could not afford to run and maintain after the grants were concluded. In addition, grants-in-aid tend to impose the same standards throughout the nation and reduce the flexibility that can result in innovative approaches to important public health problems.

Grants-in-aid had one other important effect on public health. Part of the conditions attached to grants covered the types of personnel that could be employed to carry out the programs. Many maternal and child health programs were established with federal requirements for very specific educational and experience backgrounds, including a master's degree in public health from an accredited school of public health. In fact, grants have been awarded to schools of public health by the federal maternal and child health program to train the various types of professional workers called for in the program grants to the state and local health departments.

Several important concepts emerge from this short description of the role of the federal government in public health:

1. The role of the federal government in public health was and is limited by the Constitution;
2. The role of the federal government in public health has gradually expanded, primarily due to evolving interpretations of the authority of the federal government to raise taxes to promote the general welfare and to control interstate commerce;
3. Grants-in-aid became the principal vehicle used by Congress, the president, and federal public health workers to influence state and local public health policies, programs, and employment.

HISTORY OF FEDERAL PUBLIC HEALTH ORGANIZATIONS

The federal role in public health began with the establishment of the Marine Hospital Service in 1798. With the discovery of bacteriology in France in the mid-nineteenth century came the concept of control of communicable diseases through quarantine and, later, vaccination or immunization. A series of conventions dealing with quarantine was held, beginning in Philadelphia in 1857. The fifty-four attendees discussed diseases such as typhus and typhoid, cholera, yellow fever, smallpox, and various control techniques. Similar conventions were held in 1858, 1859, and 1860, but they were interrupted by the Civil War.

The Formation of the APHA

In 1872, ten prominent men met in New York to renew the discussions. They formed the American Public Health Association (the APHA), the oldest and largest such public health association in the world. The APHA launched a campaign to form a national board of health. Such a law was passed by Congress in 1879 in the wake of yet another epidemic of yellow fever, which had entered the country through the port of New Orleans. The board had no staff. Its members were appointed by the president and included representatives from the army, the navy, and the Marine Hospital Service. Jurisdictional disputes led to its demise four years later.

The United States Public Health Service

Responsibility for quarantine control was placed in the Marine Hospital Service, since physicians were employed by the service in the major ports. By 1902, the responsibilities of the service had broadened sufficiently to cause Congress to rename it the Public Health and Marine Hospital Service and create the position of surgeon general (a military term) to direct it. (It was renamed again in 1912, shortening its title to the United States Public Health Service.)

The Public Health Service continued to grow, adding the National Leprosarium in 1917, responsible for the physical and mental examination of all immigrants that same year, and initially responsible for conducting studies and demonstrations in rural health in collaboration with the states. In 1918, a Division of Venereal Diseases was created with the power to work with the states to prevent the spread of sexually transmitted diseases. In 1929, a narcotics division was created, which subsequently expanded to become the Division of Mental Health.

The problem of child health had been a persistent concern of many individuals and groups in the United States. In 1912, Congress created the Children's Bureau and placed it in the Department of Labor. Its placement in the Department of Labor was reflective of the interest of social welfare groups and trade unions in child labor. The bureau was not empowered to engage in any direct action programs, but only to collect information and study the health and social welfare problems of children and young mothers. In 1921, with the urging of the Children's Bureau and its supporters, Congress passed the Sheppard-Towner Act, which gave the bureau authority to make grants for the express purpose of assisting the states in establishing public health programs. Largely due to opposition from the American Medical Association, the act was not renewed, and the effort ended in 1929.

The Social Security Act

But not for long. The Depression soon changed leadership in Washington, and attitudes as well. By 1935, Franklin Delano Roosevelt was successful in obtaining passage of the Social Security Act. This legislation has had a profound effect on the United States generally and on public health specifically. Title V of the Social Security Act gave the Children's Bureau (which was still in the Department of Labor) an expanded mandate to become involved in maternal and child health programs, and an initial budget of $8.17 million. It had the power to make grants-in-aid to the states and soon did so, with a network of well-trained child health advocates in key positions.

Title VI of the Social Security Act gave the Public Health Service the role of ". . . assisting states, counties, health districts, and other political subdivisions of the states in establishing and maintaining adequate public health services, including the training of personnel for state and local health work. . . ." Funds were made available for grants-in-aid and a formula was developed for dividing the money among the states. The formula was based on population, public health problems, economic need, and the availability of trained public health workers.

The Federal Security Agency

In 1939, Roosevelt, as part of a larger effort to reorganize and consolidate the work of the federal government, obtained legislation to establish the Federal Security Agency (FSA) into which, after 141 years in the Treasury Department, was transferred the United States Public Health Service. (At that time, "federal security" referred to the social security of people, not to spies and counter-espionage activities.)

The National Cancer Act

In 1937, Congress passed the National Cancer Act, which established the National Cancer Institute at Bethesda, Maryland, the offspring of the Laboratory of Hygiene at Staten Island and the first of the National Institutes of Health.

The Food and Drug Administration

In 1938, Roosevelt signed the Food, Drug and Cosmetic Act and, two years later, transferred the Food and Drug Administration (FDA) to the new Federal Security Agency. The roots of the FDA go back to the early part of the century. In his novel *The Jungle,* Upton Sinclair vividly portrayed the wretched conditions in the meat packing industry in 1906, sparking public outrage. Through the tireless efforts of Dr. Harvey Wiley of the Bureau of Chemistry in the Department of Agriculture, that public concern was transformed into the Pure Food and Drugs Act, signed by President Theodore Roosevelt in 1906. The new agency was placed in the Agriculture Department with Dr. Wiley in charge, and its responsibilities were increased by Congress over the years. The FDA, now an important part of the United States Public Health Service, employs scientists, epidemiologists, statisticians, nutritionists, chemists, biologists, and many other professional and technical health workers.

The Communicable Disease Center

During the Second World War, the Communicable Disease Center was created in Atlanta, Georgia, to deal with the spread of communicable diseases, particularly malaria, in wartime. Under the direction of Alexander Langmuir, the center developed the Epidemiologic Intelligence Service, which trained physicians in the techniques of epidemiologic investigation. These young men and women were dispatched to states, communities, and other nations to help solve some of the riddles of communicable disease and bring outbreaks under control. Still an important component of public health in the United States, it is now known as the Centers for Disease Control, and is involved in the control of noninfectious diseases, such as lung cancer and heart disease, as well as in current problems such as AIDS. In addition to epidemiologists, the centers employ laboratory workers, statisticians, educators, psychologists, virologists, and a host of other specialists in its efforts to prevent disease and disability.

Following the Second World War, the Public Health Service expanded rapidly as Congress took a more active role in shaping public health policies and programs. This willingness to intervene was shaped by two phenomena: 1) the tools for successful intervention, beginning with the great discoveries of the mid-nineteenth century, were now well understood by public health and medical research leaders, and 2) returning veterans not only accepted a governmental role in protecting their health, but they expected it. Congress passed the Hill-Burton Act, another grant-in-aid program, which made money available for the construction and renovation of the nation's hospitals. Billions of dollars were spent on more than 11,000 construction projects over the next twenty-five years, and federal standards for hospital design and operations spread throughout the nation. Ultimately, the program was partly responsible for the over-building of hospitals and led to efforts in the 1960s to control and even reduce the supply in an effort to stop the rapid increase in health care costs.

The National Institutes of Health

The National Institutes of Health (NIH), embodying the nation's enthusiasm for research and social engineering which helped it end the war, blossomed in the post-war years, with Institutes established for heart disease, diabetes, arthritis, neurological, and dental diseases. The National Institutes of Health became the largest and most prestigious biomedical research program in the world. In addition to the scientists and technicians employed on the campus in Bethesda, the NIH supports thousands of ongoing research projects in nearly every university in the country, as well as several in other nations.

The Department of Health and Human Services

In the years since World War II, the programs and responsibilities of the United States Public Health Service have expanded enormously. The various functions were reorganized in 1953 under the leadership of President Eisenhower with the establishment of the United States Department of Health, Education and Welfare. This consolidated numerous federal programs, including Social Security, the Public Health Service, and the Children's Bureau, and resulted in the largest agency in government. In terms of expenditures, it is an agency of government that is larger than most other governments in the world. The department was reorganized once again by President Carter in 1978, resulting in the establishment of a new Department of Education and the reformation of the health and welfare functions into the United States Department of Health and Human Services, known as the DHHS.

Medicare and Medicaid

A number of significant changes occurred in the 1960s during the Kennedy and Johnson administrations. Several of the important grant programs, especially those in maternal and child health, were formed into block grants. Block grants consolidated several small grant programs into a more general program to improve the health of children and offered the states more flexibility in using the money to solve problems. At the same time, Congress passed Titles 18 and 19 of the Social Security Act, known as Medicare and Medicaid, respectively. These programs were designed to cope with the fact that medical care was becoming both more essential and more expensive. On the one hand, the events of the preceding thirty years had convinced people that diseases and injuries could be treated effectively by doctors and nurses but, on the other hand, rising costs had made it impossible for a growing number of people to obtain access to these essential services.

Medicare is an insurance program for those over the age of sixty-five. Through payroll witholding taxes plus general tax revenues of the federal government, significant portions of the medical care bills of the nation's senior citizens are paid, resulting in an enormous flow of dollars into the health sector of the economy and a rapid increase in employment in that sector.

Medicare is referred to as an entitlement program. That is, citizens are entitled to the benefits of the Medicare program by virtue of their citizenship and their age. Medicaid is a federal grant-in-aid program that helps pay part of the medical care expenses of poor people. It is a welfare program administered by the states. People are not entitled to Medicaid benefits, but must apply for them and demonstrate that they are too poor to pay for needed medical care. The greatest number of beneficiaries are children and their mothers. Medicaid is the largest maternal and child health program in the nation.

Both Medicare and Medicaid have had a dramatic impact on the health care delivery system in the United States. They have affected public health activities in two ways. First, as medical care expenditures, including especially those of the Medicare and Medicaid programs, shot up from 1965 to 1981, both the federal and the state governments found themselves wrestling with health expenditures that seemed nearly uncontrollable. Many people feel that this caused the federal government to neglect public health programs, such as maternal and child health and the prevention of infectious and chronic diseases, in favor of supporting medical care efforts. By 1984, it was clear that the federal government had decreased its investments in public health and disease prevention in order to pay for its obligations in the medical care arena, and states and local governments were not able to keep up on their own.

Second, and more positively, while neither Medicare nor Medicaid was intended to pay for public health services, many state and local agencies have been successful in expanding the availability of needed services through those programs. Health departments have become much more active in organizing and providing home health services, and employing nurses, aides, therapists, and social workers. They have also expanded their work in maternal and child health as access to private care has become more difficult for low income families. Medicaid fees earned by health departments for such work have been instrumental in facilitating such developments.

THE CURRENT STATUS OF FEDERAL PUBLIC HEALTH EFFORTS

The DHHS

Currently, the United States Department of Health and Human Services is the largest federal agency with a broad and principal mission in health. Its most important parts, for purposes of this discussion, are the Health Care Financing Administration, which manages the Medicare program and the federal-state Medicaid programs, and the United States Public Health Service, which includes:

- an Office of Disease Prevention and Health Promotion,
- an Office of Health Research, Statistics and Technology,
- the National Institutes of Health,
- the Alcohol, Drug Abuse and Mental Health Administration,
- the Health Resources and Services Administration (which includes the functions of the old Children's Bureau as well as many other public health programs),
- the Food and Drug Administration, and
- the Centers for Disease Control.

Much of the work of the Department of Health and Human Services is carried on through the states and local health agencies. The department maintains regional office staffs throughout the country to oversee its programs and to assist the states. The regional offices are located in Boston (Region I), New York (Region II), Philadelphia (Region III), Atlanta (Region IV), Chicago (Region V), Dallas (Region VI), Kansas City (Region VII), Denver (Region VIII), San Francisco (Region IX), and Seattle (Region X).

The Public Health Service

The Public Health Service is staffed by both the Commissioned Corps and civil service workers. The Commissioned Corps is the present day successor to the Marine Hospital Service, and its officers hold the equivalent of military rank, and often wear uniforms. It is under the direction of the surgeon general, who does serve somewhat in the capacity of a national health officer, except that the surgeon general of the Public Health Service does not have the police power authority held by state and local health officers to control problem situations.

The surgeon general is appointed by the president and, until recently, was appointed from within the ranks of the Public Health Service. He reports to the assistant secretary of the Department of Health and Human Services. As has been seen, the scope of responsibility is vast and the number and type of personnel required to carry out the responsibilities of the Public Health Service cover virtually every category of professional, technical, and administrative worker imaginable.

Other Agencies

Several other federal agencies have important roles to play in protecting the public's health. While the Department of Health and Human Services is the only agency with a broad, overall health mission, other agencies have an important role. For example, certain agencies are responsible for the health of special groups of people, such as:

- the Administration on Aging,
- the Defense Department, which must protect and maintain the health of the army, navy, and the air force, and
- the Veteran's Administration, which provides comprehensive health services for millions of veterans.

Other agencies have a role to play in public health secondary to their primary role in dealing with other sorts of problems, such as:

- the Department of Education, which works with problems of developmental disability, health education, and teacher training,
- the Federal Trade Commission, which is responsible for

advertising and the safety of many products used daily in the home,
- the Department of Labor, which collects and analyzes important information about health status and houses the Occupational Safety and Health Administration, which is responsible for health and safety in the workplace,
- the Department of Agriculture, which, in addition to its work in pesticides, is responsible for the major federal nutrition programs such as school meals, food stamps for low income families, and the WIC program, which provides supplemental nutrition to certain women and children who are at high risk of disease due to poor nutrition,
- the Environmental Protection Agency (EPA), which is responsible for areas such as toxic wastes, air pollution, water pollution, and environmental monitoring. The EPA has derived its statutory authority through the evolution of the interstate commerce clause of the Constitution.

Finally, the federal government continues to play an important role in international health. The Public Health Service represents the United States in the present day equivalent of the Quarantine Conventions of the mid-1800s. Most of this work now takes place in the World Health Organization. In addition, the State Department includes the Agency for International Development (known as A.I.D.), which makes grants to developing nations to aid in their development of essential public health programs.

For a government without a specified constitutional role in health, the federal government has developed an extensive and important array of programs and services, including the direct provision of medical care to certain groups, major research programs, an extensive array of grants-in-aid to states to help achieve the better diffusion of what are felt to be essential and important public health services, and technical assistance and consultation to state and local public, as well as private, agencies involved in public health.

The array of talents required is mind-boggling. The personnel required runs the gamut from aviators to zoologists, from meteorologists to social workers, from physicians and nurses, to physicists and lawyers. Public health is a unique human enterprise. It does not have a single, principal discipline, but requires an interdisciplinary effort.

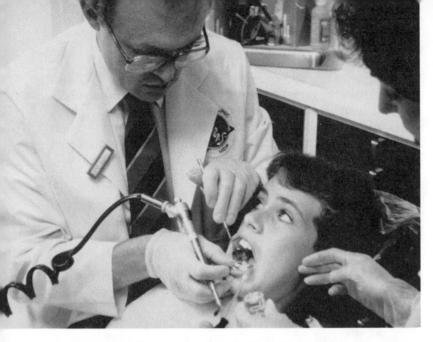

Top: This public health dentist applies protective sealants to his patient's teeth. (Department of Health and Human Services photo) *Bottom:* Epidemiologists research diseases to bring them under control and prevent their spread. (Centers for Disease Control photo)

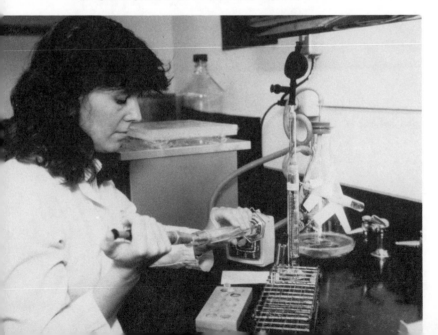

CHAPTER 5

JOB OPPORTUNITIES IN PUBLIC HEALTH

Job opportunities in public health are plentiful and varied. The majority of public health workers are found in public agencies: in health departments, of course, but also in welfare departments, education departments, environmental agencies, and other social service agencies at the federal, state, and local levels. People trained in public health are not limited to government agencies, however. Consulting firms, drug companies, insurance companies, volunteer organizations, private hospitals, private laboratories, and energy conservation firms are just a few of the businesses that hire people with public health backgrounds. Colleges and universities have a great need for public health educators and researchers. International health agencies and organizations are constantly searching for people with public health expertise.

When public health was in its infancy, the problems it dealt with were serious—the spread of smallpox, typhoid, tuberculosis, and other communicable diseases—but relatively straightforward—at least from the vantage point of the end of the twentieth century. Smallpox, once a killer at worst, a disfigurer at best, has been virtually eradicated worldwide. Vaccines have rendered polio, typhoid, and measles almost relics of the past. (Unfortunately, outbreaks still do occur, but not with the horrifying frequency that was once the case.) Clean, safe drinking water, uncontaminated food, and regular disposal of garbage and waste are things we have come to take for granted (although this situation may change if we're not careful) because of past and continuing public health efforts.

THE MISSION OF PUBLIC HEALTH TODAY

Today our world is increasingly complex and so is the mission of public health. The *Fifth Report to the President and the Congress on the Status of Health Personnel in the United States, March 1986,* published by the United States Department of Health and Human Services, describes eight major areas that will be of concern to public health going into the twenty-first century: chronic diseases; toxic wastes; behavior-related disorders; long-term health effects of hazardous chemical and physical agents; the health problems of the impoverished, disadvantaged, and migrant and immigrant population groups; new infectious diseases; the aging of America's population; and the health of infants and mothers.

Chronic Diseases

Over the past three decades the health status of the American people has greatly improved; life expectancy has increased. The surveillance of, monitoring of, and control measures for infectious diseases have paid off. As mentioned previously, many diseases that were once greatly feared have either almost or completely disappeared from the American scene, although the infectious disease control mechanisms must remain in place. According to the *Fifth Report,* public health initiatives are now ". . . increasingly directed toward preventing or reducing the incidence and severity of heart disease, cancer, stroke, accidents, premature senile dementia, neurological disorders, substance abuse, and other chronic, degenerative, and disabling disorders."

Toxic Wastes

Concern over toxic wastes is growing. So many of the everyday substances we use (plastic containers, bug spray, spot remover) are made with materials that will enter the stream of toxic wastes. We pay a price for the wonders of nuclear medicine and nuclear energy. So far no one has a good answer to the problem of disposing of radioactive wastes. The run-off of chemicals we use to fertilize our crops periodically threatens various water supplies. An oil spill at the beginning of 1988 in the Monongahela River crippled Pittsburgh for three or four days, and then other cities from Wheeling, West Virginia, to Steubenville, Ohio, as it made its viscous, destructive journey down the Ohio River. All such wastes threaten the health of human beings and the environment. Toxic wastes are not the only problem. Regular solid waste, our everyday garbage, is a problem, too. Landfills are full and it is hard to find locations for new ones. As of this writing there is a barge sailing up and down the East Coast with some of New York's garbage. There isn't room for it in its native landfill, and no one else wants it.

Behavior-Related Disorders

Behavior-related disorders are increasingly common and command more attention. Drug and alcohol abuse (referred to as substance abuse) is far too frequent an occurrence among children and young adults. The number of unintentional injuries (accidents) and suicides has risen dramatically in that population. Early pregnancy remains an important public health problem.

Hazardous Chemical and Physical Agents

Public health experts have known for a long time that certain hazardous chemical and physical agents could cause serious, noninfectious diseases. (The Mad Hatter from *Alice in Wonderland* was driven mad by the mercury he used to make hats.) The "Silicosis Blues" was written about the anguish of deadly lung disease caused by glass and sand dust. More recently, asbestos workers who worked with that mineral more than twenty years ago are now suffering from asbestosis, a debilitating lung disease caused by asbestos particles. We in America are continually searching for ways to make our lives better, safer (we think), more comfortable, and more affluent. In the process we manufacture and use chemicals and other physical substances whose long-term health effects are unknown to us. With the increased production and proliferation of these substances, questions about their long-term health effects will be studied and researched exhaustively.

Health Problems of the Impoverished and Disadvantaged

The *Fifth Report* cites the costly health problems and service needs of the "impoverished, the disadvantaged, and migrant and immigrant populations" as a major concern of public health. In their book *Public Health: Administration and Practice,* Hanlon and Pickett maintain that poverty cuts across all areas of public health:

> Poverty and a lack of education affect the biologic dimension through malnutrition and a residue of diseases and injuries that accumulate over a lifetime. It has a powerful impact on the environmental dimension as it degrades the quality of housing, increases the risk of accidents, exposes people to excessive environmental hazards such as pollutants and animate vectors of disease (rats, for example), and subjects them to excessive crowding and noise pollution. Poverty alters the behavioral dimension: the poor smoke more than the nonpoor and are less likely to value prevention highly since day-to-day survival is more of a problem. Organizationally, although the poor have a number of official support systems, they generally have poorer transportation systems, poorer schools, and less effective access to necessary health and social services. The poverty problem is so ancient and so pervasive that it . . . cannot be dealt with as a narrow public health issue, but it sets a persistent background for virtually all public health problems and programs and ultimately is the number one health problem.

New Infectious Diseases

A new generation of infectious diseases has sprung up within the past few years that requires diligent and timely surveillance, intervention, and research. The onset of Legionnaires' disease and toxic shock syndrome was cause for great alarm. The diseases are debilitating, sometimes fatal, and their causes were unknown. Through intense research and investigation, public health epidemiologists discovered the origins of both diseases, which are now usually preventable and can be treated. Unfortunately, the same cannot be said for AIDS, Acquired Immune Deficiency Syndrome. The disease is thought to be 100 percent fatal, and many public health experts predict that AIDS will remain one of the most serious public health problems, at least until the end of the twentieth century. Although AIDS affects a relatively small proportion of Americans at this time, there is no guarantee that this situation will remain stable. AIDS has reached epidemic proportions in parts of Africa. While researchers continue to search for a vaccine and treatment for this deadly disease, other public health efforts are concentrated on education and surveillance to control AIDS and stop its spread.

Problems of the Aging Population

According to the health status report, "it has been estimated that within the next 50 years more than 16 percent of the nation's population, 49 million persons, will be 65 years of age or older. Today only 11 percent of the population is in that age group. The trend is expected to lead to increased levels of chronic, long-term health problems with attendant costs, service, and management needs." We are already feeling the effects of our aging population. There are relatively fewer workers to pay into pension plans to support the health needs of older retirees. And as people get older, their chronic ailments increase; they need more care. Public health workers will need to address this problem on many fronts, from health policy analysis, to health planning, to chronic disease epidemiology.

Health of Infants and Mothers

One of our most valuable resources is our children. Although most infants and mothers receive excellent health care in the United States, there are still too many who don't. The United States has one of the highest infant mortality rates (the number of deaths of infants before their first year per 1,000 live births) among developed nations. There are too many babies born with low birth weight. Both they and their mothers often do not receive proper nutrition. Behavioral problems, chronic illness, and even mental retardation can stem from inadequate care and nutrition in infancy. Such problems can be helped with disease prevention and health promotion activities. Public health nurses, educators, and nutritionists have historically been involved in these activities. They must continue their efforts of teaching and encouraging behavioral change and work with other public health researchers and analysts to get to the underlying causes of these problems.

It should be obvious from this discussion and from preceding chapters that public health involves far more than disease or health. It is intertwined with the political, social, and economic process. Health care issues (and all health care issues are the province of public health) such as competition among health providers; regulation and deregulation; insurance benefit levels; the development and expansion of technology; ethics; law; costs and affordability; and the distribution and utilization of health care personnel, cut across all of the areas discussed. The need for effective management of human, physical, and financial resources in the study and practice of public health is essential. The multidisciplinary and interdisciplinary nature of public health gives public health workers a unique, much needed perspective on today's complex problems.

ABOUT JOBS IN PUBLIC HEALTH

Generally, the responsibilities of public health personnel include detection, assessment, and monitoring of health problems in populations; prevention of illness, disability, and premature death; health education and health promotion; control or elimination of environmental or occupational factors that result in health problems; public health administration and planning; and planning, organization, and delivery of personal health services by public health agencies.

Public health workers come from many and varied backgrounds, both health and nonhealth. Among the personnel found in public health jobs are epidemiologists, biostatisticians, general and specialized environmental health personnel, public health physicians, laboratory scientists, health agency/hospital/nursing home/long-term care administrators, health planners and policy analysts, and many other scientific and engineering personnel.

Public health people work in many different environments. For the purposes of this book, however, we will concentrate on the health department environment, both state and local, for job descriptions and salary ranges, since the majority of workers in public health are employed by public agencies. Not all public health agencies will have all the jobs described. The state and larger city/county departments have greater needs, greater resources, and hence a greater variety of positions. The smaller city and county agencies will have only selected positions and use the state agency to provide technical assistance and personnel when needed.

At this time it is possible to give only general figures as to the number of people employed in public health (although the American Public Health Association [APHA] and the United States Department of Health and Human Services [DHHS], as well as other organizations, are trying to remedy this situation). There is no reliable breakdown of numbers per job classification since each agency may have a somewhat different definition of each job classification or may call similar jobs different names. Also, public health workers are scattered among different agencies. In some states health departments are the mental health authority, the lead environmental health agency, and hospital and nursing home operators. Other states might have separate agencies for each of those functions. The multiple governmental structures involved in public health make precise enumerations of public health workers hard to come by.

Using available data, the United States Department of Health and Human Services estimates that more than 500,000 people spend a significant part of their time in public health activities. That is about seven percent of the entire health work force. Of that number, about 250,000 spend the majority of their time in public health. Of these, about thirty percent, or approximately 75,000 people, have graduate training in public health.

A 1983 study of health department personnel by the Association of State and Territorial Health Officials drew responses from forty-seven state health agencies. In that year the responding agencies employed a total of 108,100 full-time equivalent staff with a high of 15,100 in Puerto Rico (a health agency that also administers public welfare programs) and a low of 143 in Idaho. In addition to the state health agencies, there are nearly 3,000 local health departments, some employing more than 1,000 workers as in New York City, and some rural health departments employing only a clerk, a public health nurse, and a sanitarian.

Civil Service

To qualify for a job in a government agency an applicant usually must pass a civil service examination. The first state civil service law was passed in New York in 1883, and other states and the federal government soon followed suit. Today state and local civil service systems are modeled after the United States Civil Service with similar rules and regulations. Each civil service position has a job description, minimum requirements, and a salary range determined and approved by an appointed civil service commission. Although the underlying rules and regulations are similar, the specifics of civil service jobs vary somewhat from system to system. In describing the public health jobs in the following section we have used descriptions gathered from many state, county, and city health agencies to develop a common or prototypical description.

PUBLIC HEALTH CAREERS

Public health agencies employ a vast array of workers, both professional and nonprofessional, health-trained and nonhealth-trained. In a public health agency you will find lawyers, maintenance workers, secretaries, speech pathologists, licensed practical nurses, vision and hearing technicians, physical therapists, occupational therapists, statisticians, orderlies, bacteriologists, and microbiologists. The list is practically endless. Although public health departments need such personnel, they are not uniquely public health workers nor do they receive training specifically in public health. The jobs described here require public health training and/or experience or have traditionally been considered in the public health domain.

DENTAL PUBLIC HEALTH

Dental Hygienist

Qualifications: All state and local agencies require that dental hygienists receive a certificate from an approved school of dental hygiene and that they be licensed. Dental hygienists with a baccalaureate degree are sometimes eligible for more responsible positions.

Description: Dental hygienists work in either a clinical setting, such as a public health clinic, state hospital, or state correctional facility, a community setting, or a combination of two or more such settings.

In the clinical setting the dental hygienist cleans and makes a record of the condition of teeth, takes and develops X-rays, sterilizes and lays out dental instruments, and maintains patient records. He or she gives patients instructions in oral hygiene.

In the community setting dental hygienists assist in the development and operation of local school or health clinics, distribute dental supplies, develop and distribute educational materials, and make presentations to professional and lay groups about dental health, sometimes conducting in-service education programs. In some health agencies, those dental hygienists with experience and a B.A. or B.S. may administer a dental health program.

Salary range: $16,500 to $28,000.

Public Health Dentist

Qualifications: Public health dentists must graduate from an accredited school of dentistry and be licensed to practice in the state where they are employed. A master's in public health (M.P.H.) is desirable, and sometimes required, for an upper level administrative position. The M.P.H. can sometimes be substituted for a year or two of required experience.

Description: Public health dentists work in state facilities, public health clinics, or are based in the state or local health department while acting as a resource for the community.

At the entry level the public health dentist performs primarily clinical work: making oral examinations, extracting teeth, filling teeth, diagnosing and treating diseases and injuries of the teeth and mouth, constructing dentures and other dental appliances, and maintaining patient charts and histories. At this level the public health dentist may also participate in dental screening programs to identify those individuals who need dental services, give instruction in oral hygiene to residents of state facilities and/or in local clinics, and give talks and demonstrations on dental health before schools and civic groups.

In the mid-level range of positions the public health dentist has increasingly more supervisory responsibility and may become more involved in community educational, organizational, and governmental activities. Mid-level public health dentists may supervise a dental program in a state facility. At this level, the public health dentist lectures to community and professional groups and confers with government, school, health, and other social service officials on dental health matters to determine the quality of dental health care in an assigned area and the dental health needs of the community. The public health dentist also inspects dental clinics, does research on dental health issues such as caries (tooth decay) control, and promotes the fluoridation of water supplies.

In upper level positions the public health dentist is generally an administrator and planner. The public health dentist administrator directs large dental programs, sometimes the statewide dental program. That involves supervising dental clinical services through field visits; planning and supervising dental health education programs; planning and conducting dental research programs; and engaging in recruiting other public health dentists to the health department.

Future: The past few years have seen a downward trend in the employment of public health dentists in state health departments. Whether that is due to decreased hiring or a shortage of public health dentists is unclear. The job situation will vary from state to state.

Salary range: $32,000 to $61,000.

DISEASE PREVENTION AND EPIDEMIOLOGY

Epidemiologist

Qualifications: An epidemiologist must be a licensed physician, licensed veterinarian, or registered nurse with an M.P.H., or he or she must hold a doctor of public health degree or a doctoral degree with an emphasis in disease control, epidemiology, and/or public health programming.

Description: Epidemiologists are the detective/scientists of public health. The public health epidemiologist designs, plans, and/or directs the survey, investigation, reporting, and control of diseases and injuries to determine those factors responsible for the distribution of those diseases and injuries in the population. The epidemiologist then may establish and manage programs to identify, test, and treat other potential victims. Examples of such diseases and injuries include typhus, AIDS, rubella, rabies, hepatitis, Reyes Syndrome, botulism, motor vehicle accidents, suicides, falls, fires, Legionnaire's disease, lung cancer, and toxic shock syndrome.

Epidemiologists coordinate specialized disease prevention programs, such as rabies immunization of animal control workers and students, to give health assistance to those in areas of critical disease exposure. They also develop and maintain an ongoing data bank of the characteristics and statistics of disease among population groups. They develop policies and procedures to be followed in epidemiological investigations, including specimen collection, diagnosis verification, animal quarantine, and statistical analysis.

Epidemiologists write articles and give speeches and demonstrations about various aspects of epidemiology and disease control. They advise the public, medical professionals, hospitals, and other concerned organizations about appropriate public health services and treatment for specialized public health problems.

The epidemiologists in public health agencies must have many talents and skills. They must not only possess a thorough knowledge of statistics, the biological sciences (e.g., physiology, anatomy, biochemistry), sociological factors as they relate to disease communication and control, and public health administration, but must also be able to deal effectively and clearly with a variety of individuals and agencies from lay citizens to veterinarians, physicians, and administrators.

Future: Epidemiologists are in demand in a growing number of areas. Within the past few years epidemiology as a way of analyzing a problem has led to its use in a wide variety of studies: the epidemiology of aging, the epidemiology of obesity, even the epidemiology of health services administration. Epidemiologists who study noninfectious diseases and trauma of environmental and behavioral origins probably will be in particular demand. Jobs for epidemiologists are expected to increase in traditional public health agencies, research institutions, educational institutions, private industry, and overseas.

Salary range: $35,000 to $60,000.

Public Health Consultant

Qualifications: A baccalaureate degree from an accredited college or university and a master's degree in public health or related field such as nursing, nutrition management, genetics, or speech audiology are required for public health consultants.

Description: Public health consultants are usually found at the state and federal levels. They provide technical assistance to local health agencies by making on-site visits and helping plan, implement, and evaluate health care programs. The public health consultant also meets with private organizations to assist in designing health care programs and procedures and helps coordinate the work of local agencies in delivering needed health care services. The public health consultant designs training programs, develops and updates procedures manuals, and develops criteria for evaluating health care program services.

At upper levels the public health consultant is responsible for supervising lower level consultants and is in charge of larger, more complex health care programs. He or she coordinates activities in the field with those of the central office.

The public health consultant must have a thorough knowledge of public health programs and practices, good organizational skills, and must be able to deal effectively with a variety of people.

Salary range: $23,000 to $42,500.

Public Health Field Worker

Qualifications: A high school diploma with some college or office experience is required for the entry level position. For upper level positions a baccalaureate degree is necessary. A master's degree in public health will substitute for some experience.

Description: At the entry level the public health field worker surveys public health programs, assists in the orientation and supervision of part-time personnel in those programs, and participates in health promotion activities with physicians, civic groups, rural organizations, and school organizations toward the goal of improving the health of the community.

At the upper level the public health field worker identifies and evaluates those elements used in successful health program development. He or she establishes close working relationships with other governmental agencies to obtain good health and educational programs for private industry, nursing schools, and local health departments. The public health field worker develops methods for hard-to-reach groups and maintains a good relationship with the media.

Salary range: $9850 to $28,000.

Public Health Investigator

Qualifications: A baccalaureate degree with a major in the social, natural, or behavioral sciences is required. At the upper level an M.P.H. is desirable.

Description: The public health investigator usually does field work in locating, preventing, and controlling sexually transmitted diseases through investigation, treatment, and educational services. He or she interviews infected patients and their contacts in an effort to locate the source of disease and refers them to local clinics for treatment. The public health investigator maintains regular contact with private physicians, laboratory personnel, and state and local health department personnel to improve case reporting and remain current on treated cases and diagnostic techniques. The investigator also keeps physicians informed as to the status of the sexually transmitted disease problem in their area.

At the upper level the public health investigator assumes a supervisory role, supervising local health departments regarding methods of dealing with sexually transmitted diseases, and training lower level investigators. The upper level investigator has responsibility for a larger geographical area, does field work, and provides educational services to prevent the spread of the more serious sexually transmitted diseases, such as AIDS and chlamydia.

Besides having a thorough knowledge of sexually transmitted disease and public health practice methods, it is essential that the public health investigator be a tactful person who is able to maintain confidentiality.

Salary range: $13,000 to $33,200.

ENVIRONMENTAL HEALTH

Sanitarian Aide

Qualifications: The only requirement for a sanitarian aide is a high school diploma.

Description: The sanitarian aide, under the direct supervision of a sanitarian, performs routine inspections of facilities, runs tests on consumer products, and reports violations of environmental laws or regulations. He or she explains health department policies and regulations to those affected by them.

Salary range: $9000 to $20,000.

Sanitarian

Qualifications: Sanitarians must have a baccalaureate degree with an emphasis on the natural or biological sciences. Some health departments will accept a combination of some post-secondary work, training, and experience, but the B.S. is preferable and makes advancement easier. Most states require that sanitarians be registered by the state or the National Environmental Health Association.

Description: In civil service classifications sanitarians are usually divided into beginning, senior, principal, and administrative levels. They are sometimes called environmental specialists, environmental scientists, environmentalists, or given a programmatic name, such as vector control inspector. Such titles usually refer to public health sanitarians.

At the beginning level, general sanitarians perform inspections and investigations of such facilities as food service establishments, food processing plants, and food distribution facilities to determine their compliance with environmental health laws and regulations. They investigate complaints involving possible sanitation law violations and prepare reports with recommendations for corrective measures and follow-up investigations. Beginning sanitarians also inspect public and private facilities such as schools, motels, hotels, and recreation areas, checking food protection, water supply, waste disposal, lighting conditions, ventilation, fire safety, cleanliness, and animal or insect vectors of disease, such as mosquitoes and rats. They also inspect operational aspects of swimming pools, small untreated water supplies (wells), and sewage disposal facilities.

A beginning sanitarian in a specialized program may participate in the inspection of larger facilities or systems, such as air pollution sources, water supply systems and plants, industrial and domestic waste treatment systems, and solid and hazardous waste management systems. He or she participates in field investigations and epidemiological studies of environmental hazards, assists in monitoring air and water quality by gathering and interpreting data, and collects samples of air, water, and/or waste for bacteriological, chemical, or biological analysis. Beginning sanitarians also compile and process information for construction permits, or approvals for sewer and wastewater treatment facilities. They may participate in a special investigation of unusual environmental problems with representatives of other state agencies and confer with officials, owners, and operators of industrial and domestic waste treatment systems with regard to laws, regulations, and requirements of the environmental program.

In the upper levels sanitarians have increasingly more responsibility and deal with more complex technical problems, such as the inspection of nursing homes and related facilities that are subject to complex state and federal regulations and standards. At this level the public health sanitarian serves as a liaison with other agencies, organizations, and industries and offers technical assistance to ensure compliance with environmental health laws. He or she also may be the director of a small health department at this stage.

The administrative progress of the sanitarian is highly structured, especially in state and large city/county health agencies. At the supervisory and administrative levels, the sanitarian may first direct one program at the district level, then head the coordination of several programs, then finally be responsible for all of the environmental programs in one district, or be responsible for one program, such as milk sanitation, food service sanitation, or food, drug, and cosmetic labeling, statewide. On rare occasions a sanitarian may become the state director of environmental health.

Besides having a thorough knowledge of the principles, techniques, and practices of environmental sanitation, the sanitarian must be able to interact well with people. In some communities the sanitarian, along with the public health nurse, is the most visible representative of the public health agency.

Future: Environmental health is the fastest growing area in public health. Employment opportunities for sanitarians remain very good, especially for those with advanced technical training and degrees. There are many jobs available for public health sanitarians. Unfortunately, salaries are not in line with the training and expertise of the upper level sanitarian. Until that situation changes, there will probably be a shortage of public health sanitarians.

Salary Range: $19,000 to $41,000.

Engineering Technician

Qualifications: Engineering technicians are required to have an associate degree in engineering technology from an accredited college or university, and a baccalaureate degree in engineering, mathematics, or the natural sciences from an accredited college or university for the advanced level.

Description: The engineering technician performs technical work assisting engineers in the areas of air and water pollution, surface mining and reclamation, sanitary engineering, and environmental health and utility engineering. At the beginning level the work involves the collection and analysis of air and water samples, conducting field inspections of mining and utility sites, performing mathematical calculations, data collection, and chemical analysis.

At the more advanced level the engineering technician evaluates air and water pollution permit applications and surface mining permit applications, performs engineering calculations, and designs and prepares technical reports on observations from field inspections and laboratory analyses.

Salary range: $15,000 to $30,000.

Public Health Engineer

Qualifications: Public health engineers must graduate from an accredited college or university with a baccalaureate degree in engineering (civil, environmental, chemical, sanitary, or mechanical), and for upper level positions a master's degree in engineering and/or public health is desirable. Registration as a professional engineer is usually required by the state.

Description: The public health engineer oversees and directs the performance of a variety of environmental engineering activities to protect and improve land and water resources and the air quality to maintain a clean, healthful environment.

At the beginning level the public health engineer assists senior engineers in surveillance, inspection, and investigation of environmental systems, including public water supply or waste water treatment systems, air quality control systems, industrial or solid waste collection and disposal facilities, or facilities producing, processing, or using radioactive material. He or she performs routine engineering calculations and collects environmental samples for bacteriological, chemical, biological, and radiological analysis.

The beginning public health engineer also is involved in the evaluation of facilities operation.

Mid-level engineers provide guidance and technical assistance to consulting engineers, public officials, municipalities, and industries in preparing and revising plans for the construction or modification of the previously mentioned facilities, and then review the plans and specifications to determine compliance with local, state, and federal regulations and standards. They also perform field inspections and surveys of environmental quality control facilities for evaluations in the areas of design, efficiency, and pollution assessment, and they provide technical assistance and training to operators of sanitary landfills, air quality control systems, solid waste disposal systems, industrial waste sites, and/or operators of water and waste water treatment plants. They do engineering design work for environmental quality control devices, systems, and facilities and interpret and advise industry and the general public about environmental laws, regulations, and policies.

Upper level engineers perform similar tasks with more supervisory and governmental responsibility. For instance, they coordinate and direct the engineering activities for the planning, construction, and operation of the systems and facilities previously mentioned. They also analyze applications for federal and state construction grants and advise municipalities of funding sources for construction of environmental systems and facilities. The upper level public health engineer researches engineering programs and staff requirements in order to make recommendations for changes in policies and procedures.

At the administrative level the public health engineer directs lower level engineers in the operational aspects of engineering programs, such as air pollution control or facilities management, and in their reviewing capacity. He or she provides consultation to engineers on unusual or complex engineering problems and directs studies and surveys on environmental health hazards. The administrative engineer coordinates with other state and federal agencies and districts in the implementation of construction programs for environmental quality control and makes recommendations for changes in statutes and regulations concerning environmental quality control. In a few states, an environmental engineer is eligible to become state health director with the required experience and a master's degree in public health.

Future: Highly trained public health environmental engineers are in great demand by both public health agencies and private industry. Besides their knowledge of engineering, their understanding of environmental rules and regulations is invaluable in both the public and private sectors.

Salary range: $22,500 to $53,000.

Industrial Hygienist

Qualifications: A baccalaureate from an accredited college or university in industrial hygiene, engineering, or the physical or biological sciences is required.

Description: The industrial hygienist investigates working conditions at places of employment, often industrial worksites, to identify hazards that may cause disease or injury and determine their source. He or she takes samples of work materials to detect and evaluate employee exposure to toxic substances, uses ventilation testing equipment and special measuring devices to determine airflow rates, noise, lasers, and other physical factors in the workplace, and measures airborne concentrations of dust, gases, and mists using air sampling instruments and collection devices. Industrial hygienists prepare reports covering their findings and propose corrective measures that comply with governmental health rules and standards. They also consult with management, industrial engineers, employee representatives, and other agencies concerning industrial health problems and their solutions.

Upper level industrial hygienists have supervisory, and sometimes administrative, responsibility. They coordinate and evaluate the work of other industrial hygienists, are involved in program planning, conduct in-service training programs in industrial hygiene, and assess industrial hygiene needs in their region. They also coordinate their activities with other departments and help develop policies and procedures related to industrial hygiene, sometimes providing direction and administration of a statewide industrial hygiene program.

Future: With hazardous substances proliferating in the workplace, there is an increasing demand for well-trained industrial hygienists.

Salary range: $17,500 to $50,000.

PUBLIC HEALTH EDUCATION

Public Health Educator

Qualifications: A baccalaureate degree from an accredited college or university with a major in health science, community, or public health education is preferred. A master's degree in public health is desirable, and is sometimes required, for positions above the entry level.

Description: The public health educator is usually based in the health department. He or she is responsible for working with health department staff, community agencies, professional groups, schools, and the general public in organizing community health resources and disseminating health information materials, conducting promotional campaigns, and stimulating interest in the improvement of the health practices of the public. The public health educator also conducts surveys to find out about the attitudes and behavior of individuals toward health problems, identifies community health resources and the leadership available to assist with health problems, establishes needs and goals for public health education programs, and trains local health department staffs and volunteers in the methods, practices, and purposes of health education. The public health educator selects, prepares, and uses brochures, news articles, poster exhibits, and television, radio, and slide show scripts in organized health education efforts. Public health educators also sometimes work in specialized programs, such as family planning and chronic disease control.

Upper level public health educators have increased responsibility in planning, coordinating, and directing health education programs. If they are employed at the state level, their geographical area of responsibility will grow larger to encompass regional, then comprehensive statewide programs. At this level public health educators assess regional and statewide needs and resources in health education, and they evaluate and offer consultation and assistance to local health agencies.

Public health educators need extensive knowledge of health education techniques, organization methods, communication skills, and group dynamics, and must be familiar with statistical methods and with the behavioral modifications that motivate individuals to change their behavior to improve and maintain good health.

Future: As is the case with public health dentists, the trend is for fewer public health educators to be in state health departments. Whether this is due to health educator shortages or to changed hiring practices in health departments is unclear. However, health educators do appear to be employed more often in the community and in the hospital or clinical setting. Patient education has become more common with current efforts to reduce the length of time a person stays in the hospital. The current emphasis on improving one's health through changing lifestyles has led to jobs for health educators in businesses and organizations in the private sector.

PUBLIC HEALTH MANAGEMENT

From the descriptions of the many jobs it is evident that many management and administrative positions in public health agencies are achieved through expertise and experience in a particular profession. The entry level sanitarian, through hard work, increasing expertise, and years of experience, becomes the director of the statewide food sanitation or milk inspection program. The public health dentist who begins his or her career in a clinic works up to being director of the division of dental public health. The same progression holds true for public health nurses, nutritionists, and physicians.

But public health problems are more complex today than they once were. Health agencies have increasingly complicated responsibilities. The director of disease control must attend to designing studies, analyzing data, and implementing disease prevention strategies; there is often not enough time to properly perform the administrative functions required to run a health program or division successfully. The health managers described below perform those vital administrative functions. Trained specifically in public administration and/or public health, these managers are in ever greater demand by public health agencies and by hospitals and other health organizations in the private sector. The positions listed below represent only a small sample of the managerial positions available in public health. Each agency has its own structure and will have its own titles.

Program Representative

Qualifications: A program representative is required to have a baccalaureate degree from an accredited college or university.

Description: The program representative promotes and helps accomplish the goals of a specific health program. Activities include integrating new employment programs into the health care system; planning and conducting investigations into individual and community health problems; monitoring, correcting, and approving reports from local agencies in accord with state and federal regulations; and training new employees.

Salary range: $14,000 to $25,000.

Program Specialist/Evaluator

Qualifications: A baccalaureate degree from an accredited college or university is required for the lower level positions. For upper level positions, a master's degree in public health, public administration, business administration, or a related area is required.

Description: The program specialist/evaluator works in programs ranging from disease investigation, to nutrition, to health education. The program specialist/evaluator provides technical assistance in program planning to divisions within the health department by analyzing management and financial information, and by analyzing the division's data base to determine its clients' health status and the effectiveness of its delivery systems. The specialist/evaluator directs research activities to improve statistical data collections, and establishes uniform procedures and standards of operation.

On a higher level the program specialist/evaluator is involved in the planning, financial administration, and personnel management of a highly specialized program. He or she may also be involved in negotiating with federal agencies for grant support.

Salary range: $17,500 to $35,000.

Training Coordinator/Director

Qualifications: Either a baccalaureate from an accredited college or university, or a master's degree in business administration, public administration, sociology, psychology, or a related field is required.

Description: The training coordinator determines the manpower and training needs of the public health agency, then plans and implements programs to meet them. He or she conducts workshops to promote staff development; offers technical assistance and consultation in developing training programs for staff members; assists in developing new training opportunities in colleges and universities; coordinates orientation, staff development, and in-service training activities; and designs evaluation systems for training programs.

The training director supervises the training coordinator. He or she also organizes and develops training manuals; tests and evaluates training procedures, multi-media visual aids, and other educational materials; coordinates and establishes training courses with technical and professional courses offered by community schools; and develops the annual budget for the training program.

Salary range: $19,000 to $37,000.

Public Health Administrator

Qualifications: A public health administrator must have a baccalaureate degree from an accredited college or university for assistant positions; a master's in public health, public administration, or business administration is needed for upper level positions.

Description: Public health administrator positions include administrative assistant, deputy director, assistant director, and administrator titles. They generally involve assisting in the formulation of departmental policies and procedures, developing budgets, assisting in development of legislation, overseeing and monitoring contracts, and other responsible administrative duties. The scope of duties of the public health administrator will differ from program to program.

Salary range: $20,000 to $49,000.

PUBLIC HEALTH NURSING

Many nurses who are not public health nurses work in a health agency. They are clinical nurses who work in state hospitals, correctional institutions, and sometimes clinics. Their duties are no different from those of nurses found in any other settings. The following positions are specific to public health.

Public Health Nurse

Qualifications: A diploma from an accredited school of nursing is adequate for some entry level positions. Many public agencies require a baccalaureate degree in nursing for entry level as well as higher levels. For upper level supervisory or administrative positions, a master's degree in public health, nursing, or nursing education is often required. A license to practice in the state of employment as a registered nurse is mandatory.

Description: Public health nurses provide nursing services in homes, clinics, schools, and other community settings. They are generally involved in health department programs for child health, maternity care, family planning, general communicable diseases, and sexually transmitted diseases. Much of the work of the public health nurse centers on health education. During home visits, besides providing skilled nursing care to patients, the public health nurse develops nursing care plans, and provides health supervision, counseling, and teaching to patients and their families. In addition, he or she (usually she, but there is a growing number of male nurses) participates in community education programs, gives direction to community health workers, and performs physical assessments of patients and screens for specific diseases at various clinics.

At the next level, the public health nurse assumes a supervisory role, sometimes supervising a nursing staff in a public health department, or supervising a specific public health program, or serving as the only nurse in a small county health department. Here the public health nurse can perform specialized, complex nursing services requiring advanced training and/or experience. Some public health nurses become involved in regulatory activities at this level, evaluating nursing services as part of a team that licenses and certifies health facilities. Besides evaluating the quality of nursing care, the public health nurse might also evaluate the use of prescription and nonprescription medicines, observe kitchen personnel, check menus and equipment, and observe sanitary conditions and practices, all of which are important in the care of patients. At this level, too, the public health nurse becomes involved in the planning and establishing of clinics, community health education programs, and in-service training for nursing and other health department personnel. She also acts as a liaison between the health agency and other community or governmental agencies.

In the upper levels the public health nurse can go in several directions. She can become the director or manager of progressively larger, more complex nursing programs either geographically or programmatically. That is, she may be responsible for the operation of many programs (e.g., maternal and child health, communicable disease screening, or school health) in a small geographical area, or for a specialized program covering a large area, a district, several counties, or the entire state. (Those public health nurses involved in specialized programs are sometimes certified nurse practitioners; they receive additional training in a specialty.)

Having administrative responsibility for a program means being in charge of planning, formulating policies and procedures, preparing budgets, preparing reports for other officials, managing personnel, assessing program needs and ways to meet them, and serving as chief liaison with the community and other departments and agencies to explain the activities and purposes of the program. Those public health nurses directing specialized programs often function as nurse consultants. In the larger city/ county agencies, and in some state health agencies, it is possible to advance to being the overall director of nursing.

Future: It is difficult to predict future needs for public health nurses, but at this time good, trained public health nurses are in demand.

Salary range: $18,000 to $43,000.

Public Health Nurse Consultant

Qualifications: A master's degree in nursing, public health, or a related field and state licensure as a registered nurse are required.

Description: At the beginning levels the public health nurse consultant assists local health departments and private health care facilities in developing, establishing, implementing, and maintaining professional nursing care programs. This involves providing information and guidance in the development of policies and standards of nursing practice for new programs; offering consultation and technical assistance to individuals, institutions, and agencies through on-site visits and workshops; visiting facilities to see that standards for accreditation and certification are being met; identifying program needs and evaluating programs; and conducting and participating in conferences, institutes, and workshops with other agencies and associations concerning health care problems, solutions, and resources.

At upper levels the public health nurse consultant assumes progressively more supervisory and administrative responsibility in a nursing care specialty area (e.g., pediatrics, or infectious diseases) or in areas such as health education or licensure. In this capacity she meets with department heads and citizen groups on nursing and health care issues; plans, designs, and carries out various nursing programs, projects, studies, and research; and gives program direction in administration, practice, education, and research. She also helps program and service directors determine health policy and procedures for operating good programs.

At the highest level in a state agency, as well as her statewide administrative responsibilities, the public health nurse consultant allocates nursing resources throughout the state, participates in developing and monitoring federal and state legislation related to nursing, develops and promotes general standards of nursing care, designs and directs statewide research programs relating to nursing and health care programs, and plans and directs the provision of nursing consultative services to local health departments, clinics, and hospitals.

Salary range: $23,000 to $42,000.

PUBLIC HEALTH NUTRITION

Public Health Nutritionist

Qualifications: A baccalaureate degree from an accredited college or university with major studies in foods and nutrition or closely related areas is required for entry level positions. For upper level positions a master's degree in public health nutrition or foods and nutrition is necessary. Most public health nutritionists must also be registered as a professional dietitian by the American Dietetic Association.

Description: Public health nutritionists provide technical and advisory services to local health departments and related community agencies. In that capacity they counsel patients in public health clinics about therapeutic diets and provide counseling to people with specific nutritional problems. They provide information and advisory services to staff members in public health clinics and to teachers, social workers, and community groups; conduct classes on nutrition and consumer education for patients, with emphasis on nutrition of pregnant women, infants, and children, and provide training for institutional food service personnel; and survey and evaluate institutional food service operations.

At the upper levels, public health nutritionists develop nutrition education materials, and provide nutrition education programs for clients in food preparation, consumer education, weight control, and related areas. They also plan and conduct surveys and studies to assess nutritional problems in geographical areas, and use the results as a basis for program and nutrition education development and to evaluate the change in nutritional behavior of individuals or groups after participation in nutrition programs. The public health nutritionist at this level maintains cooperative relationships with personnel of related agencies in order to coordinate program activities and goals.

As with other public health professionals, the public health nutritionist, with the proper education, training, and experience, is able to advance to the administrative level. There he or she plans, directs, and supervises comprehensive and specialized nutritional programs and serves as a dietary consultant on administrative and technical problems related to nutrition in group care and other state-run facilities.

Future: The *Fifth Report to the President and Congress on the Status of Health Personnel in the United States* stated that there is a great need for nutritionists trained in public health, especially those trained at the doctorate level, to work in educational and research institutions and in senior positions in nutrition units of health agencies. Citing the study "Public Health Nutrition: A Review of the Field and Training Programs" by J. E. Brown, the report said that "demand for public health nutritionists has remained strong because of the need created by health, nutrition, and food assistance programs and services provided by public and private agencies." That includes such programs as health services for handicapped children, the special Supplemental Food Program for Women, Infants, and Children (WIC), and nutrition programs for older Americans. Positions for public health nutritionists also seem to be growing in private health care delivery organizations as health care expands from hospital-based to community-based systems. The growing interest of Americans in improving their health through exercise and nutrition has increased the demand for nutrition information in the mass media and has increased the number of positions in settings such as physicians' offices, fitness centers, and worksite health promotion programs.

Salary range: $16,500 to $35,000.

PUBLIC HEALTH PHYSICIANS

Public Health Physician—Clinical

Qualifications: Graduation from an accredited medical school or school of osteopathy is necessary; often residency training and/or board certification in a specialty are required. Licensure to practice medicine in the state where the physician is employed is mandatory.

Description: The clinical public health physician, sometimes called a public health clinician, medical officer, or another title, is engaged primarily in providing direct medical services in a public health clinic. Or, at a higher level, a public health physician develops and supervises diagnostic and treatment programs for a large specialty public health clinic or for all clinic activities in a designated health district or area. In this capacity, besides examining patients and diagnosing their disorders, the public health physician is responsible for the medical direction of community health services, supervises and directs the activities of employees of a local health department, cooperates with public and private agencies in the development of community health programs, is a medical consultant to local health department personnel, and enforces health laws and regulations.

At the higher level the clinical public health physician conducts follow-up studies of more difficult cases, directs a district-wide or statewide program for the prevention and control of specific medical problems, establishes standards, policies, and procedures for the program, and cooperates with federal, state, and local agencies in planning new programs, conducting consultations on specialized medical problems, and participating in research and pilot projects conducted by such groups.

Salary range: $31,000 to $75,000.

Public Health Physician—Administrative

Qualifications: Graduation from an accredited school of medicine or osteopathy is required. A master's degree in public health or board certification in preventive medicine is desirable, and often required, in this area.

Description: The administrative public health physician differs from the clinical physician in that most of his or her activities deal with health administration rather than the direct delivery of medical services, although the public health physician-administrator must have a thorough knowledge of the principles and practices of modern medicine. The public health physician serves as the health or medical director of community health departments, combined health districts, statewide public health programs (such as programs in epidemiology or maternal and child health), or the deputy director or director of the state or local department of health. In this role public health physicians are known by titles such as medical director, medical program director, medical officer, public health officer, health director, or health commissioner (there may be others).

In this capacity the public health physician plans, promotes, and supervises community health services in designated areas, including programs in the prevention and control of diseases, health education, maternal and child health, and environmental health programs. He or she surveys area health needs, evaluating the effectiveness of programs in meeting those needs; coordinates health department services with those of other agencies and private practitioners; provides medical consultation services to private practitioners, lower level health officers, and other officials; and establishes policies, procedures, and evaluation mechanisms for program services. The administrative public health physician keeps informed of financial resources available from state, federal, and other agencies for special programs or services that would benefit the community, district, or state; manages the budget; reports regularly to the appointed board of health on department operations, needs, and recommendations; meets regularly with division directors to determine if objectives are being met and to make changes if necessary; and directs research and investigation into public health problems. The public health physician in this capacity also maintains close contact with community service organizations, local, state, and federal agencies, professional organizations, and the media to coordinate and promote public health services; he or she directs the enforcement of all state public health laws.

The knowledge and skills necessary to be a successful public health physician-administrator are many and varied. Besides having a thorough knowledge of the principles and practice of modern medicine, a public health physician must be knowledgeable about public health theory and practices: the laws, codes, and regulations pertaining to public health and related areas and the principles and practices of public administration. He or she also must have the ability to work effectively with officials of other agencies, employees, and the general public.

Future: See the discussion of public health physicians in chapter 7.

Salary range: $42,000 to $90,000.

PUBLIC HEALTH PLANNING AND ANALYSIS

Health Planner

Qualifications: A master's degree in public health, public administration, or health planning is required.

Description: The health planner is involved in studying and administering programs to develop needed health resources and in planning and evaluation. At the upper administrative level the health planner is responsible for the coordination, development, and writing of the broad, comprehensive, departmental public health program plan (planners at a lower level work on researching and writing specific areas of the plan), and updates and publishes it annually. The planner also develops evaluation mechanisms of all new health programs; is responsible for the identification and application of government and nongovernment funding resources that could be beneficial to the public health agency; monitors all contracts and develops all subcontracts; provides consultation and technical assistance to department professionals and representatives of community-health related programs; and is responsible for statistical analyses of factors relating to health care issues.

Future: See the discussion about health planners and policy analysts in chapter 7.

Salary range: $25,000 to $42,000.

PUBLIC HEALTH SOCIAL WORK

Public Health Social Worker

Qualifications: A baccalaureate degree from an accredited college or university with a major in social work or the behavioral sciences is required for entry level positions; a master's degree in social work is usually required for upper level supervisory/administrative positions.

Description: At the beginning levels the public health social worker provides social work services to children and adults in public health agencies, through clinics, and in state facilities such as hospitals and institutions for the developmentally disabled. The social worker conducts interviews and obtains information in other ways from clients, families, teachers, ministers, social agencies, and other relevant sources to identify social, economic, emotional, health, or physical problems; determines need and eligibility for such services as aid to families with dependent children, food stamps, day-care and nursing home assistance; refers clients to appropriate programs and does follow-up; and assists clients in utilizing available community resources. The public health social worker investigates suspected cases of abuse; provides for protective and support services for the abused or neglected; counsels families on proper care; may need to testify in court; and coordinates with social agencies, hospitals, clinics, and other community resources in attempting to meet client needs. At this level the public health social worker also locates and inspects child care facilities prior to licensing and inspects them periodically to assure that licensing regulations, procedures, and standards are met.

At the intermediate level positions, public health social workers handle the more difficult, complex cases that require extensive professional diagnostic and treatment expertise. They also assume a supervisory or consultative role, supervising and assisting lower level social workers with difficult cases and coordinating the assignments of caseloads. Public health social workers at this level develop and maintain working relationships with agency and community resources and act as liaisons to the community, explaining the role of social work to the public and to medical and nursing student groups.

At the upper administrative levels the public health social worker is in charge of a social work program of moderate to large size and complexity, depending on his or her experience and capability. Here the social worker coordinates the social work program with available community resources and establishes and maintains cooperative relationships with other public and private agencies; directs social work in-service staff development programs; ensures compliance with federal, state, and agency regulations; and confers with medical staff and department heads on professional problems and assignment of work.

Future: There is a demand for social workers, especially on the planning and management levels.

Salary range: $14,000 to $33,500.

Public health careers are challenging, complex, and rewarding. The salaries and job descriptions discussed above are not exact. There is often an overlap in responsibilities; what the public health nurse consultant does in one agency the director of nursing services will do in another. Nutritionists, sanitarians, physicians, and nurses are all involved in health education efforts, not just health educators. Salaries vary widely from agency to agency, setting to setting; those quoted above are typical, although there are instances of salaries above and below the ranges listed.

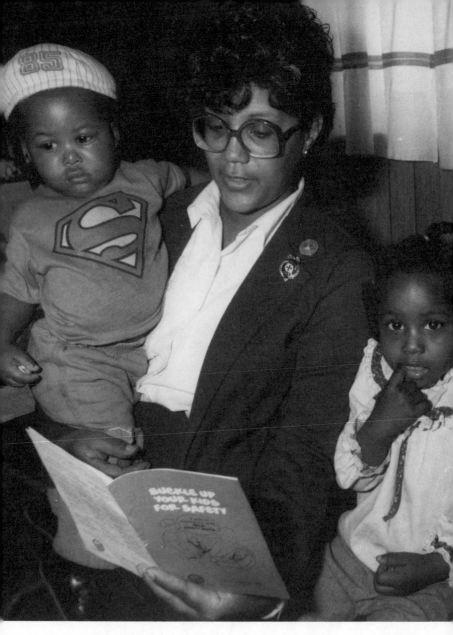

A public health nurse uses a picture book to teach children about safety.
(Chicago Department of Health photo)

CHAPTER 6

WOMEN AND MINORITIES IN PUBLIC HEALTH

The concerns of public health are the concerns of all United States citizens. All of us are threatened when an epidemic occurs; most of us know of someone who was killed in a car accident involving a drunken driver; almost all of us have been vaccinated against polio, measles, diphtheria, and other serious diseases. (Until recently, we were all vaccinated against smallpox, but public health workers have succeeded in eradicating the disease from the world. The last known case was reported on October 26, 1977, in the seaport town of Merka, Somalia, on the horn of eastern Africa. We know that this disease is at least 3,000 years old from the discovery of smallpox lesions on the body of the Egyptian pharoah Ramses V. The eradication of smallpox, which has taken many lives over the centuries, is one of the greatest triumphs of public health.) Our drinking water and the food we eat are made safe through the sanitation efforts of public health.

There is another concern of public health that is the concern of us all: the health and welfare of the poor and disadvantaged. The financial burden of caring for the poor and disadvantaged is heavy. But the waste of precious human resources that poverty produces is far costlier. In today's complex, competitive world we cannot afford to lose the potential talent and creativity of that too-large segment of society.

From its earliest history in the United States, public health has

91

directly served those left out of the mainstream of society. The Marine Hospital Service was established soon after the United States won independence to care for merchant sailors who otherwise would not have been cared for. Lemuel Shattuck, in his monumental report written in 1850, outlined the special needs of the poor. Public health programs for mothers, infants, and children are generally targeted to the poor and minorities who often do not have the education, resources, and access to good medical care that the majority of people in the United States has.

The public health commitment to serve women, minorities, and the disadvantaged is mirrored in a similar commitment to those groups in education and employment. Women and minorities are both strongly encouraged to enter the many varied careers available in public health. The opportunities are there.

WOMEN IN PUBLIC HEALTH

Women traditionally have played a leading role in public health. Public health nurses and public health nutritionists, primarily women, have had positions of leadership and responsibility since the beginning of the twentieth century. Few women in any other profession, with the possible exceptions of nursing, teaching, and drama, attained comparable status at that time. Although health directors at the local and state levels were usually male physicians, public health nursing directors served as managers of one of the two largest components of the agencies (the other being environmental health).

Public Health Nurses and Nutritionists

Public health nurses work in the community and in homes. Their role is very different from a hospital nurse's, who works directly under a physician's supervision with strict rules to follow. The public health nurse has to make decisions on her own, often quickly, in emergency situations that are often potentially devastating, such as a young and inexperienced mother's early care of a developmentally disabled child. She has to be competent, self-reliant, and adaptable. With her responsibilities and experience in the field, the public health nurse is a mainstay in the running of local health departments, and her input is essential to the effective management of larger local and state health departments.

As part of a bureaucracy, the public health nurse, and also the nutritionist (programs in nutrition are basic to maternal and child health), run programs and departments. They report to the health director, but they are responsible and independent in their own right.

Over the years the scope of health departments has expanded. Trained public health nurses are as important as ever. With nursing as a base, they can branch off into such fields as health administration, epidemiology, or health education. Nutritionists are in greater demand than ever before. Not only are they necessary in health department programs, but there is a crucial need for nutrition researchers and faculty members at colleges and universities.

The Children's Bureau

At the federal level, the Children's Bureau, which was concerned with the health and welfare of children, was established in 1912 during the presidency of Theodore Roosevelt. The first chief was a woman, Julia Lathrop. She was quoted in the November, 1912, issue of the *American Journal of Sociology* as saying, "This bureau was first urged by women who have lived long in settlements and who by that experience have learned to know as well as any person in the country certain aspects of dumb misery which they desired through some governmental agency to make articulate and intelligible." Although the bureau originally was in the Department of Commerce and Labor (its primary advocates were those concerned about child labor), it served a public health function: to promote the welfare of mothers and children. This bureau, supported by women's organizations, often administered by women, and staffed by women (men supported and participated in this bureau, too, but its driving force came from women), had a profound effect on subsequent health policy and health care legislation at the national level.

Other Roles

Two other fields in which women predominate have gained importance: health education and public health social work. As people assume more responsibility for their own health care and maintenance, they need knowledge that the health educator can provide about health, self-care, and how lifestyle and behavior affect health. The public health social worker works in both institutional and community settings, counseling clients and coordinating the services they need.

Women have had leadership roles in public health for some time, but those roles have been in traditionally "women's" professions. Physicians, engineers, sanitarians, epidemiologists, biostatisticians, and health directors have generally been men. That situation has begun to change.

The Future for Women in Epidemiology

Epidemiologists have, until recently, usually been male physicians. In the past few years many more women have entered the field. Some public health experts think the change may have occurred because the focus of epidemiology is changing and growing.

The main focus of epidemiology used to be the study of infectious diseases: how they developed, how they spread, and how to control and/or prevent them. Although infectious diseases from AIDS to chicken pox are still with us, they are no longer the threat they once were. AIDS is extremely serious, but so far it affects a relatively small proportion of the population; many children might get chicken pox, but compared to AIDS, it is usually not a very serious disease. This contrasts sharply with the many deaths or debilitated lives that used to occur as a result of contagious diseases such as scarlet fever, tuberculosis, diphtheria, and polio. Until the late 1940s it was not uncommon for at least one member of a family to be affected by one of these diseases. Polio was still a major health threat until the mid-1950s, when the Salk vaccine came to be widely used. (The Salk vaccine was given as a shot with a booster a year or so later; several years later the Sabin polio vaccine was developed, which could be dropped onto a sugar cube and swallowed, a sweet way to prevent polio.)

The care of infectious diseases was the province of physicians, who were predominantly male. (Most physicians still are male, but the number of female physicians has practically quintupled in the last twenty years.) In the past ten years, however, the study of noninfectious chronic diseases, such as arthritis, heart disease, and cancer, has become a major focus of epidemiology. Such illnesses involve not only medical care, but also behavioral changes, learning how to cope with long-term disability, and self-care regimens, women's traditional areas of responsibility. Other areas of epidemiology are also growing: the epidemiology of aging, the epidemiology of health services administration, and the epidemiology of obesity. For whatever reason, an increasing number of women are epidemiologists. With the current and future need for highly trained epidemiologists, there is room for many more.

Women as Health Administrators and Planners

Two other areas in which women are very prominent are health administration and health planning and analysis. An approximately equal number of men and women are involved in both fields. Men are more often affiliated with hospitals, while women tend to work in government agencies as consultants and educators in these specialties. At this point, given the complexities of the health care system in the United States, there are many job opportunities for competent health administrators, male and female.

The job situation for health planners is somewhat less clear. Some public health experts predict that the demand for health planners will grow as it becomes increasingly apparent that there are no easy solutions to the problems of the American health care system. Recent attempts to contain soaring health care costs seem to have failed; there are still far too many people without access to adequate health care, and allocation of resources is an ongoing problem. Should the next million dollars be spent on a new infant intensive care unit, or should it be spent on intensive family planning programs aimed at preventing the birth of babies who need intensive care? If, as predicted, more health planners are needed, women are in a good position to fill those roles.

Women in public health have begun to make substantial inroads in upper level leadership and policy-making positions. A growing number of health director positions at the state and local levels, positions once held only by male physicians and occasionally male engineers or sanitarians, are now held by women. Women frequently fill positions as deputy directors and assistant directors, too. Several factors could be responsible for this change. Many health directors, especially at the state level, are required by law to be physicians, and there are more female physicians than ever before. Social and political barriers to women in leadership positions have lessened somewhat in the past few years. Most health directorships are political appointments; governors and boards of health may not be as reluctant to appoint a woman to important, policy-making positions as they used to be.

Perhaps most important to the elevation of women to upper level leadership roles is the general receptivity to women in public health. Women traditionally have held responsible positions in health departments and have been central to their operations. Although health directors are still predominantly men, women are playing increasingly prominent roles in public health.

In most environmental health jobs the number of women still lags far behind the number of men. Engineers and sanitarians have traditionally been men and still are. At this point, though, women would be gladly accepted in these areas in schools of public health. (In some health departments, especially smaller, rural ones, there may be resistance to women in these positions, but they would be welcome in most health departments.) Women are already visible participants in industrial hygiene programs. They also are hired as biostatisticians, toxicologists, microbiologists, and as other much needed scientists and researchers.

For women, public health is a field of great diversity, challenge, and opportunity. More than fifty percent of students in graduate schools of public health are women at this time. This is particularly encouraging in a field that requires a high degree of expertise and training in almost all areas. In public health careers women will find a level of equality and advancement opportunity unusual in many professions. Public health is committed to serving the needs of women, both as clients and as practitioners.

MINORITIES IN PUBLIC HEALTH

People often speak of minorities as if the same statistics and conditions hold true for all minority groups. That is not the case. Each minority group has its own culture, its own identity, and its own strengths and weaknesses. According to the 1980 census of population, 20.1% of the population of the United States is comprised of what is at this time considered to be racial or ethnic minority groups. This racial minority population is made up of black Americans (11.5%), Hispanics (6.4%), Asians and Pacific Islanders (1.5%), and American Indians, Eskimos, and Aleuts (0.6%). (We will refer to Asians and Pacific Islanders as Asians; American Indians, Eskimos, and Aleuts as American Indians.)

Minorities in Health Professions

Of these minority groups, blacks, Hispanics, and American Indians are considered to be underrepresented in the health professions. That is, the percentage of these minorities in health professions (e.g., doctor, dentist, epidemiologist) does not correspond to their percentage in the population as a whole. For example, although Hispanics are at least 6.4% of the United States population, only 2.0% of dental school graduates in 1982 were Hispanic.

If these groups did not want to enter the health professions, it would not matter that they are underrepresented. But the health professions are attractive to many people. They offer prestige, relatively high incomes, and are interesting and rewarding. The fact that there is such a low percentage of blacks, Hispanics, and American Indians in most of the desirable health professions indicates that these groups are unable to get the necessary education and training to enter these professions.

The situation with the Asian Americans is quite different. Although they are a minority group, they are more often overrepresented in the health professions. In 1982, Asian Americans made up 2.9% of the graduates of medical schools in the United States. That percentage may seem low until you remember that Asian Americans make up only 1.5% of the United States population as a whole. The percentage of Asian American medical school graduates is almost two times higher than their percentage in the general population.

The commitment of public health to the underprivileged, disadvantaged, and minority groups is very basic. Public health clinics, public health hospitals, maternal and child health programs, substance abuse programs, mental health clinics, and other programs serve the needs of everyone, but they have a special mission to serve the disadvantaged who often have nowhere else to go for their health care needs. Minority health workers are badly needed in public health to meet the needs of the client groups.

Minorities in Public Health Education

As is the case with women, the commitment to minorities as clients is reflected in the commitment to minorities in public health education and employment. Schools of public health actively seek out minority students; in some cases they are successful, sometimes not. There is no doubt that they want more minority students than they presently have.

Over the years the trend has been for schools of public health to have a higher percentage of minority graduates than other graduate schools in the health professions. Even so, blacks and Hispanics are underrepresented in both the student bodies and the faculties of the schools. The lack of enrollment of black students in schools of public health is a particularly distressing situation. (Although Hispanics are also underrepresented, they are not as severely underrepresented as black students.)

The mid to late 1970s seems to have been the high point for black graduates from schools of public health. Since then black enrollment and the number of black applicants has gone down, despite major efforts to recruit black students. No one is sure why this is so. Possible reasons for the decline may be the rising costs of education, the lack of scholarships because of decreases in federal funding, and the increased necessity to rely on loans.

The major barriers to minorities in public health, particularly blacks and Hispanics, seem to be the reasons cited, as well as the lack of access to a good public school education, an essential prerequisite to higher education, and certainly a prerequisite to most careers in public health.

Public health careers are definitely open to minorities because minority practitioners are desperately needed. Those people from minority groups who do enter the field of public health often attain policy-making and leadership positions. As with women, the opportunities for minority workers in public health are easily demonstrable. But unlike women, the underrepresented minorities, especially blacks and Hispanics, need to be encouraged to enter schools of public health in far larger numbers.

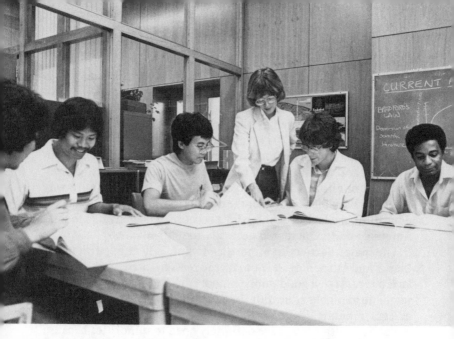

Top: The important characteristics of public health education are the study of epidemiology and public health policy. (UCLA School of Public Health photo by Norm Schindler) *Bottom:* Training to become a nurse includes practical work experience as well as coursework. (Cedarville College photo)

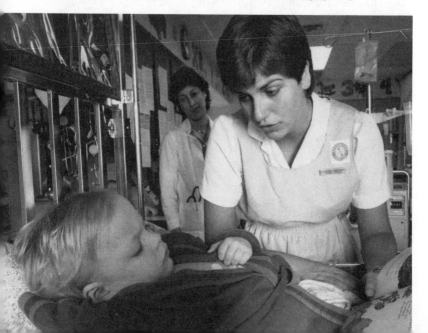

CHAPTER 7

EDUCATION FOR PUBLIC HEALTH

Education for a career in public health is straightforward in some respects, but made complicated by the unique nature of public health programs. Public health requires many talents, so virtually any career training can be suitable—as a secretary, accountant, nurse, meteorologist, engineer, lawyer, social worker, dietitian, librarian, or painter. Health departments have need for some or all of these, depending on the nature and scope of the services provided by the agency.

Public health programs need people who have "clinical" skills—the sorts of capabilities found in the general community. People to fill teeth, type reports, paint walls, and examine healthy babies are all necessary. In this context, a clinical skill is the ability to perform a specific task requiring specific training. But a career *in* public health, rather than simply working in a public health agency, entails skills requiring training beyond clinical skills. For example, working as a painter in a hospital run by a city health department is not really a career in public health.

Public health workers, whether technical, administrative, or professional, need skills that can often be acquired outside of public health education programs, but these skills should be coupled with public health training.

THE UNIQUE CHARACTERISTICS
OF PUBLIC HEALTH EDUCATION

The important characteristics of public health education are the study of epidemiology and an understanding of when, why, and how a public agency ought to intervene in the affairs of a community, a family, or an individual.

Epidemiology

Epidemiology is the study of the characteristics of a disease or injury as it occurs in population groups. This is quite different from the study of disease in a clinical training program such as medicine or osteopathy, nursing, psychology, or dentistry. Epidemiologists must either understand, or work with others who do understand, the way in which a disease or injury evolves, its diagnosis, its complications, and its treatment. But more importantly, they need to know why some people get the disease (or are injured) and others do not. It is the purpose of the epidemiologist to help find ways to prevent the spread of a disease or, if that is impossible, to reduce its severity. Why are fat people more likely to develop diabetes than thin people? Why are black people more susceptible to high blood pressure than white people? Why do cigarette smokers generally have shorter lives than nonsmokers, and why do some cigarette smokers not develop lung cancer (a more difficult question)? Why do teenagers have such a high rate of death due to accidents (now known as "unintentional injuries") and other forms of violence?

Answers to such questions help scientists better understand the mechanisms involved in such diseases, and they help people design programs to reduce their incidence or severity.

The skills involved are quite different from those that make a good physician in a clinical practice setting. Most people, when they think they may have a disease, are not interested in the probability of having a particular disease, but rather in whether they have the disease. Do they have it or don't they? It's a yes-or-no question or, in the binary world of computers, an open or shut gate, a 1 or a 2. It would help you little if your physician said that you had one chance in forty-seven of having colon cancer. The question is whether you do, and what can be done about it. Later on, you and other members of your family may be interested in why the disease occurred (or didn't), and whether anyone else in the family has an increased risk of developing the same problem and what can be done to reduce that risk, but when a person is suffering from a disease, it is not a good time for such speculation.

The opposite is also true. When public health agencies are trying to understand why some adult males have a diphtheria bacterium in their throats and others in the same community do not, a practicing physician is not the best person to answer the question. Physicians in clinical practice see primarily sick people. They tend to view the community in a skewed or crooked fashion. A pediatrician who sees thirty children in a day, ten of them with colds, may think that one-third of all children have colds. But for every child who came to the physician's office, there are ten others who did not (some of whom, by the way, do have colds), making the true rate of illness something more like three percent, or one out of every thirty.

A home owner may be concerned about a failing septic tank system because the sewage is backing up in the pipes, causing an unpleasant living situation. A plumber may be called in to correct the problem. An environmental health worker may tell the home owner how to get the problem corrected, but he or she is primarily concerned about the potential hazard to the community's water supply.

Public Health Policy

Equally important is the study of public health policy. Why has a governmental presence in health been organized in every community of the country? Under what circumstances will society tolerate or even insist on governmental intervention in what would otherwise be considered a private matter?

While many parents become fiercely involved in arguing about what can and cannot be taught to their children in schools, most of them accept without question the authority of the school system to require that the children be immunized against certain diseases before they can enter school.

While people argue vociferously about their right to eat whatever they please, communities insist that restaurants be inspected by environmental health workers.

While we protect the right of people to reject medical care if they wish to, we insist that people with certain diseases be either treated or isolated from the rest of the community.

While people insist on the right to privacy and the right to take risks with their own lives, most states now have laws requiring the use of seat belts in cars.

When, why, and how should a public health agency intervene? These are not scientific questions. Their answers are to be found through the study of history, philosophy, ethics, law, administration, and political science. While public health programs are not the only places where people can find out about such decisions, those decisions are an integral part of the public health discussion. The study of public health policy is not so much a matter of learning skills or memorizing facts as it is the experience of debate and discussion.

VALIDATING EDUCATION

Many careers in public health involve licensure, certification, or registration. It is useful to understand the difference. (The true public value of such concepts is another matter—a very complicated one, and beyond the scope of this book.)

Consumers want to know something about the quality of a product or service. In most cases, quality can be judged by the buyer. In some situations, however, that is difficult, and an unsafe practitioner can be dangerous. It is one thing to get a bad haircut, but quite another to have a bad kidney operation.

Accreditation

As consumers, we are interested in the competency of a service provider. That, however, is often very difficult to measure. One substitute for a direct measurement of competency is evaluation of the provider's training. Most public, and many private, schools voluntarily subscribe to an accreditation process. Accreditation (to bring credit to something) involves a careful review of the educational program to see if its curriculum, its resources, and its faculty are adequate for the stated goals of the program. It can be assumed that someone who graduates from an accredited program has at least been exposed to a satisfactory educational experience and has earned an acceptable grade. Many agencies (schools, health departments, and hospitals, among others) insist that an applicant must have completed an accredited program of training or education in order to be eligible for a job. But it is the educational program, not the candidate, that is accredited.

Certification

One way to judge the competency of individuals to perform tasks is to test either their knowledge or their ability to do them. Certification is a voluntary act that uses written, oral, and performance tests to judge competency. To be eligible for certification, a candidate usually must have completed successfully an accredited or approved program of study. A physician may graduate from an accredited medical school and later apply for certification as a specialist. Such certification is a voluntary action. Some hospitals will not allow physicians to perform certain procedures unless they have been certified by the appropriate specialty organization. Certification represents a "seal of approval." It is usually awarded by others who have specialized in the same field. Certification is an attempt to evaluate the person.

Registration

Under certain circumstances, legislatures have passed laws establishing registration procedures. It should be pointed out that registration (and licensure, which will be discussed next), while it involves legislation, rarely is the result of a public concern for safety. Laws supporting registration (and licensure) are usually the result of lobbying by the professional group. Whether that lobbying is to protect the public from unqualified people, to reduce competition, or to increase prestige is a hotly debated question. Whether registration (or licensure) really protects the public is also a hotly debated question.

Registration requires the successful completion of a training program or some other form of experience. The successful applicant is registered and entitled to use the term *registered* (nurse, sanitarian, or well digger, for example). Unregistered people can practice the trade (if they can get a job or customers), but cannot call themselves registered. In states where registration systems are in effect, civil service systems often specify, as a condition of being eligible for a job, that the applicant must be registered.

Licensure

The apex of competency evaluation procedures is licensure. As is true of registration, licensure is an act of government. Unlike registration, however, licensure restricts the practice of the act, as well as the name or title. Licensure involves a finding by the state that a certain service is both essential to health and welfare and potentially dangerous if performed by an unqualified person. The state forbids people from performing the act, and then, by examining people who have graduated from accredited programs, the state grants a license to do what would otherwise be illegal. The license is given because there is an assumption that if the applicant can pass the test, he or she is sufficiently competent to be safe— not necessarily good, but safe.

While still often referred to as registered, nurses must be licensed to practice nursing. Originally they obtained recognition of registration from the state (beginning in 1900). Subsequently, beginning in 1938, nursing was successful in attaining the stature of licensure.

Legislative bodies are increasingly wary of proposals to establish new licensing programs. Professional groups, on the other hand, are zealous in their pursuit of licensure. Again, whether the motivation is based on concern for the public's welfare, or simply the welfare of the professional group, is difficult to determine.

Many careers in public health involve one or more of the above competency validation procedures: completion of an accredited program of study, certification by professionals in the same field, and registration or licensure. It is not clear that this will continue. There is some pressure for other forms of competency validation. If the purpose of such testing is really to judge competency, what difference does it make how the applicant became competent? If an interested person can master brain surgery at home and prove his or her competency, why worry about the accreditation of the program with all of the administrative problems and costs that accreditation involves? If a laboratory can produce accurate results, why worry whether the technicians are certified or registered or, in some states, licensed? It is the result that counts.

For the time being, however, people interested in a professional career in public health, as in many other fields, should pay special attention to the requirements for work in their chosen field and the availability of accredited education and training programs.

GENERALIZE OR SPECIALIZE?

To repeat what has been said many times before, public health is a unique field. While there are twenty-three graduate schools of public health in the United States, there is not a single discipline of public health similar to the disciplines of law, medicine, music, or architecture. The graduate schools or programs provide separate training programs for epidemiologists, biostatisticians, administrators, environmental health workers, toxicologists, health educators, and others. Public health depends on the successful blending of many skills or disciplines. Yet who is to manage such an effort? A specialist, or someone with a broad, general knowledge of public health policy, epidemiology, and administration?

Public health, as is true of other demanding careers, provides individual rewards (salary, recognition, and title, as well as job satisfaction) for people who have special skills. But the most important tasks of the future will require an interdisciplinary approach—the ability to work across traditional organizational boundaries: AIDS, alcohol-related problems, aging and dependency, maternal and child health. Each requires the contributions of specialists with the ability to function effectively in a broad effort organized to achieve not an individual, but a group, goal. While knowledge and information are expanding so fast that specialization is necessary for the successful performance of many tasks, the future requires successful generalists who can define problems, formulate policies, and organize the work of specialists to attain a socially determined goal.

It would be difficult to define a successful educational program for a public health generalist, but the role is clearly there for those who find satisfaction in the outcome.

EDUCATIONAL PROGRAMS FOR PUBLIC HEALTH CAREERS

As indicated earlier, public health careers involve a mixture of clinical skills (dentistry, mathematics, environmental sciences, and so forth) coupled with public health knowledge. The two aspects of training may be acquired in different settings.

Frequently people enter public health work with a background in one of the clinical skills, and later return to school to study public health as they make more permanent career choices. Alternatively, the two types of training for public health can be acquired simultaneously in a public health educational program, such as in one of the twenty-three accredited schools of public health, or in one of the public health or preventive medicine programs located outside of schools of public health, such as a health education program, a program in general community health, or a medical school department of preventive medicine. (See Appendix D for a list of currently accredited schools and programs providing public health education.)

For detailed information about any of the careers described, write to the appropriate organization listed in Appendix A.

Dental Public Health

Most of the personnel in dental public health work are involved in one of three activities: 1) clinical dentistry for certain target population groups, 2) fluoridation or other programs designed to prevent dental disease, or 3) dental health education. The professionals involved usually combine clinical education in dental health, such as dentistry or dental hygiene, with education in public health. The clinical education is most often acquired in a dental school. An undergraduate degree (either a B.A. or a B.S. is required) is followed by two or more years of education and training in a professional school. Following that, a minimum of one year is needed in either a school of public health or in a community health education program.

At this time, four schools of public health provide specific training in dental public health at the master's level: the Harvard University School of Public Health, the School of Public Health at the University of Michigan, the School of Public Health at the University of North Carolina at Chapel Hill, and the School of Public Health at the University of Alabama at Birmingham. These programs offer either a combined program with the dental school, or specific training oriented toward dental public health issues and programs. Doctoral level training is available for those who wish to pursue a research or academic career in dental public health.

Disease Prevention and Epidemiology

There are very few training programs in disease prevention at this time, but more programs may be developed over the next few years. Generally, public health careers in disease prevention follow training in a specific field, such as dental public health or health education. The School of Health at Loma Linda University, however, offers master's and doctoral level training designed to prepare individuals without specific clinical training for work in certain areas of disease prevention and health promotion.

In a more general sense, careers in disease prevention and health promotion develop from a background in epidemiology or health education. Training in epidemiology, generally available only through schools of public health, prepares people for work in disease surveillance, program planning, and the design and implementation of specific disease prevention programs, both for infectious diseases such as AIDS, and for chronic diseases such as cancer, heart disease, diabetes, or arthritis. It is common for people to specialize in a particular area. The educational programs are at the master's level. Doctoral level training is also available in many schools of public health for those who may have an interest in research and teaching. It is likely that an increasing number of people with both master's and doctoral level training will be needed in the years ahead as state, local, and federal public health agencies concentrate increasingly on the prevention of common and serious diseases.

Undergraduate education is relevant to a career in epidemiology, but usually not sufficient. A background in the biological sciences with some mathematics and psychology or other social and behavioral science would be especially useful, although majors in the humanities and social sciences can be very effective for those who go on to graduate level training. Health departments do employ people with only undergraduate level training for work in disease prevention programs, such as immunization programs and disease investigation (such as programs to combat sexually transmissible diseases), but graduate level training is necessary for career progression beyond the entry level or administrative support roles.

Graduate training usually requires two years of work. Some schools offer a master's degree after only one year, but such programs are often limited to those with other graduate degrees (such as medicine, nursing, or environmental health) or several years of experience.

Another discipline often coupled with epidemiology, although it is very different, is biostatistics. Biostatistics involves the collection and analysis of numerical information relating to biological phenomena. The number of people not wearing seatbelts killed in automobile accidents, how many smokers contract lung cancer, and how many obese people suffer from high blood pressure are examples of some of the questions biostatisticians study. They generally work closely with epidemiologists, providing the statistical framework needed to examine hypotheses in epidemiological studies. Training in biostatistics is generally available only through schools of public health and preventive medicine programs in medical schools, although statistics, as a branch of mathematics, is taught in agriculture, business administration, and engineering. Graduate training requires one or more years of work, depending on the requirements of the program, prior training, and the degree sought.

Environmental Health

Educational and training programs for careers in environmental health are increasingly diverse, as the field has taken on added importance in recent years. Until the 1960s most environmental health workers were either sanitarians or engineers. Sanitarians usually require at least a college education. Sanitary or environmental engineers usually require postgraduate training in public health or in sanitary engineering.

In recent years, the field has exploded as state and federal programs in both air and water pollution control have developed, and the nation's attention has been directed to the enormous problems of waste disposal. New careers in environmental epidemiology, toxicology, and risk assessment have developed rapidly with high level training programs in many schools of public health, as well as in chemistry departments, physics, and engineering.

The Bureau of Health Professions in the United States Public Health Service has estimated that there are about 30,000 environmental health workers with 20,000 sanitarians, 6,000 industrial hygienists, and 4,000 in research and teaching. Many more will be needed in the years ahead.

A career as a sanitarian (often referred to as an "environmental health worker" or "environmentalist") can follow an undergraduate educational program with an emphasis on the biological and natural sciences. Many states now register sanitarians, and only those who are registered are eligible for employment in an official public health agency. The National Environmental Health Association (NEHA) offers registration for sanitarians who have an appropriate baccalaureate degree and experience in a general environmental health program, for environmental health technicians who do not have a baccalaureate degree but do have some experience, and for hazardous waste specialists who have a baccalaureate degree and three or more years of experience.

NEHA registration as a sanitarian requires successful completion of a standardized examination, or registration by a state program with comparable education, testing, and experience requirements. A baccalaureate degree from a college or university with a curriculum that has been approved by the National Accreditation Council for Environmental Health Curricula, or a degree in biology, chemistry, physics, sanitary engineering, or other discipline, with thirty semester hours of science and college algebra, plus two years of experience, is required. Registration as an environmental health technician requires a two-year degree in environmental health or a related field.

NEHA publishes self-help, self-paced learning modules that can help prepare people for registration. At the present time, undergraduate programs in environmental health accredited by the National Accreditation Council for Environmental Health Curricula can be found at the following institutions:

California State University at Northridge
California State University at Fresno
Colorado State University at Fort Collins
University of Georgia at Athens
Boise State University in Idaho
Illinois State University at Normal
Indiana State University at Terre Haute
Eastern Kentucky University at Richmond
University of Massachusetts at Amherst
Ferris State College at Big Rapids, Michigan

Mississippi Valley State University at Itta Bena
Montana State University at Bozeman
East Carolina University at Greenville, North Carolina
Western Carolina University at Cullowhee, North Carolina
Bowling Green State University at Bowling Green, Ohio
East Central State University at Ada, Oklahoma
Oregon State University at Corvallis
East Tennessee State University at Johnson City
Brigham Young University at Provo, Utah
Old Dominion University at Norfolk, Virginia
University of Washington at Seattle
University of Wisconsin at Eau Claire.

Since the requirements for registration accept many other degrees, entry into the field can be obtained from almost any accredited college or university, but the above programs have sufficient interest and expertise to have pursued the subject of environmental health in an organized fashion.

Many engineering schools provide education and training in environmental health. Schools of public health provide both master's level and doctoral level training.

In general, those interested in a career in environmental health should obtain a baccalaureate degree with a major in environmental sciences, the biological sciences, or the natural sciences, and should consider acquiring master's level training in public health if they are interested either in an environmental health specialty or in program management.

Health Education

The field of health education has been divided into three different specialties in the past few years: community health education, school health education, and health education in medical care settings. A fourth specialty in the occupational setting is emerging. Health education in medical care settings is involved in educating patients in order to improve their recovery and reduce long term disability. This field, presumed by many to become increasingly important as the nation attempts to make its medical care system more efficient, as well as effective, will not be discussed here. Those interested should contact individual graduate level programs to find out whether that specialty is covered.

It is easy to become confused by the nature of health education programs. Every state has one or more colleges or universities that train teachers for careers in the school system. Most of these programs offer courses in health education, and some offer a complete training program. These are not the same as health education programs in schools of public health that focus more on the behavioral sciences and have community groups as their focus. School health education programs are concerned more with classroom education, curriculum design, and school health issues. Education and training in community health education, either in one of the schools of public health or in one of the accredited programs in community health education, will not prepare someone for a teaching career in most public education systems, and vice versa.

Undergraduate programs in community health education are numerous and can serve as an entry point for the career. However, graduate training in an accredited program is desirable for people who wish to progress beyond the entry level into program planning, design, implementation, and management.

Graduate programs in community health education are accredited by the Council on Education for Public Health. The Council accredits both schools of public health and a number of programs in community health education outside of schools of public health. The Society for Public Health Education has an approval process for baccalaureate degree programs in community health education.

At the present time, there are more than 140 undergraduate programs in health education, 91 master's level programs, and 36 that offer a doctoral degree. Of course, not all of these are in community health education.

Management in Public Health

Historically, most public health managers (health officers, directors, and others) had a background in a clinical area, such as nursing, medicine, or environmental health, and became either program directors or agency directors by virtue of their acquired experience and often the successful completion of a master's program in public health. That is still considered to be the preferred route to a successful career in public health administration.

With the increasing complexity and the expansion of technology in the health sector generally, and in public health policy specifically, people trained in management are needed both at the local and state levels to cope with the planning, organization, and ongoing management of disease prevention and health promotion programs. Generally speaking, lacking a clinical background, such work requires graduate level training in public health administration.

There are several routes to education for a career in public health management that can be followed. Most schools of public health offer master's level training in public health administration. In addition, there are a number of programs in health services administration that are accredited by the Accrediting Commission on Education for Health Services Administration (ACEHSA) that are located outside of schools of public health. (ACEHSA also accredits programs in health services administration that are a part of a school of public health.) Such programs are often found in schools of business or schools of public administration.

An alternative to a master's degree from a health services administration program is a dual degree involving graduate training in public health (M.P.H.), and either business administration (M.B.A.), or public administration (M.P.A.). For a number of reasons, such training, which usually takes two and one-half to three years of full-time study, has some significant advantages. The entire field of public health, including prevention, medical care, and environmental health, has become increasingly complex. It requires a physician seven to eight years to become a sufficiently well-trained practitioner. It should not come as a surprise to find that those who are responsible for managing important public health programs would be required more than a one-year training program after college to become successful. The public health degree tends to be a knowledge-based degree with an emphasis on epidemiology and health policy, while the M.B.A. or M.P.A. degrees are skill-based degrees, providing the student with the techniques needed to manage.

Nursing

Nurses comprise the largest single group of public health workers. They are involved in management, planning, regulatory activities, health education programs, disease prevention programs, and home health nursing.

Current estimates indicate that more than 400,000 nurses will be needed in community health work in the 1990s, with twenty-five percent of those trained at the graduate level and the rest at the baccalaureate level.

Traditionally, most nurses in the United States were graduates of diploma courses that required two to three years of training and experience. In recent years, however, the profession has determined that a baccalaureate degree is the necessary level of training required for entry into the field. Given the increasing complexity of health care programs generally, and the level of public expectation, this seems a desirable step.

There are some other points of controversy, however. How to distinguish nursing in general from public health nursing particularly, and questions about generalization versus specialization have continued to provoke intense debate within the field.

Undergraduate education programs in nursing exist in every state. Only a few of them offer a specialty program in community or public health nursing, although most offer one or more courses dealing with some of the special features of such activities.

While popular attention often centers on the highly trained nurse in a sophisticated hospital environment, public health nursing is, in many ways, more demanding and more rewarding. In the hospital environment, sophisticated protocols have been developed to guide actions and responses to emergency situations, and a variety of other specialized workers is available to assist in dealing with complex situations. In the community setting, however, the nurse must often react to very complex problems with no such protocols available and no backup specialists. Helping a new mother cope with what may turn out to be a developmentally disabled child during a home visit can have a permanent effect on the mother's relationship with the child and on the child's well being. That's the demanding part. The rewards come from the successful management of such complex situations as an independent health professional.

In small towns and rural counties, nurses without a baccalaureate degree or special training in public health can be employed and work effectively, especially if there is a support structure available either within the community or in collaboration with the state health agency. In larger communities, however, a baccalaureate degree is often required for work as a public health nurse. For those who wish to become supervisors or program managers, master's level training is necessary, either in nursing or in public health.

Nutrition

Ideally, public health nutrition requires both clinical training in human nutrition and training in public health. Many nutritionists in public health agencies do not have both.

There are about 3,000 master's level nutrition positions in state and local health departments. Another 2,000 are needed to meet the demands. Currently most public health nutritionists work in the WIC program, a state program funded almost entirely by the United States Department of Agriculture. Others work with senior citizen groups or other organizations that may have special needs. Only a few public health nutritionists work in exclusively clinical settings where they deal with individual patients with nutritionally-related diseases.

Public health nutritionists should pursue registration as a registered dietitian (R.D.), since most jobs require such certification. Registration requires the successful completion of a course of study acceptable to the American Dietetics Association and an examination. (Note that in this case the term *registered* is incorrectly used, since it is the private act of a voluntary association rather than the official act of a state board or agency.) For those who are interested in nutrition program planning and management, a master's degree in public health nutrition is desirable. Such training programs include course work in epidemiology, biostatistics, community planning, and public health practice, as well as nutrition and the behavioral sciences.

The field of public health nutrition began in the 1920s with the development of federal and state maternal and child health programs. The first graduate programs were initiated in the 1940s with initial standards developed in 1950. These are periodically updated by the Association of Faculties of Graduate Programs in Public Health Nutrition in collaboration with the Association of State and Territorial Directors of Public Health Nutrition. In 1985, there were approved programs in nineteen universities, most of them in schools of public health.

Approved Programs in Public Health Nutrition

University of California at Berkeley*
University of California at Los Angeles*
Case Western Reserve University, Department of Nutrition,
    Cleveland, Ohio
Columbia University, Teachers College, New York
Cornell University, Division of Nutritional Sciences, Ithaca, New York
Harvard University*
University of Hawaii*
Loma Linda*
Massachusetts Institute of Technology, Department of Nutrition and
    Food Science
University of Michigan*
University of Minnesota*
University of North Carolina at Chapel Hill*
Pennsylvania State University, College of Human Development, State
    College, Pennsylvania
University of Puerto Rico*
University of Tennessee, Collect of Home Economics, Knoxville
University of Toronto, Faculty of Medicine
Tulane University*

Virginia Polytechnic Institute and State University, Department of
  Human Nutrition and Foods, Blacksburg
Eastern Kentucky University, Department of Home Economics, Richmond
Southern Illinois University, Department of Food and Nutrition,
  Carbondale
*in a school of public health

In addition to these, several other universities offer programs in nutrition that would qualify graduates for registration.

Physicians

Physicians are badly needed in public health agencies, as clinicians, program planners, managers, and in regulatory activities. The basic education is, of course, graduation from an accredited school of medicine or osteopathy.

Physicians are needed for clinical work in pediatrics, obstetrics, family practice, general internal medicine, and psychiatry.

In addition, there is a serious shortage of physicians with training in public health and public administration who can analyze and form policy, develop and manage programs, and direct public health programs and agencies. Those interested in such careers should pursue a master's degree in public health as well as a clinical degree. In some universities, it is possible to pursue a master's degree in public health (or in community or preventive medicine) and a degree in medicine or osteopathy simultaneously. It is also possible for physicians to enter a residency training program in preventive medicine. Such programs qualify residents for board certification in general preventive medicine and public health. Requirements are completion of the clinical doctoral degree, one year of supervised clinical training in an approved program, one year of academic work, usually in a school of public health or a department of preventive medicine in a medical school, and a year of supervised experience in a preventive medicine setting. At the end of the seven years, successful graduates have a doctoral degree in medicine or osteopathy and a master's degree in public health, and are eligible to take the examination that qualifies them as specialists in preventive medicine and public health.

Planning and Analysis

State health agencies, large local health departments, and federal public health programs need well-trained planners and program analysts. During the 1960s, several degree programs were developed in public health planning, but the concept has not been successful, and most such educational programs now involve a more sophisticated curriculum centering around areas such as economics, resource allocation, systems analysis, organizational behavior, the law, and political science.

Such curricula can be found in several schools of public health. They are also available through a school of public health in collaboration with schools of business or public administration or in public policy programs. It is possible to enter the field with only a master's degree in business or public administration, but the work really requires exposure to and experience in public health policy analysis and formation, including epidemiology and biostatistics.

The field is not well-defined at the moment, but it is growing in importance, especially at the state level, where responsibility for complex programs such as medical care for the poor, long-term care, and maternal and child health is placed. Several schools of public health now offer a specific concentration in public health policy.

Social Work

Nearly half of all social workers in a survey carried out by the National Association of Social Workers in 1982 said that they were involved in public health social work: 18.1% in medical or health care; 26.5% in mental health; and 2.9% in substance abuse or alcoholism work. Most of the social workers in public health agencies are involved in maternal and child health programs.

As is true in all areas of public health, there is a need for people with social work training both in clinical settings and in community health settings working as planners and managers. While some of the clinical work can be carried out by social workers with undergraduate degrees, career development requires graduate level training, including a master's degree in social work (M.S.W.) and, often, an M.P.H. degree as well.

Most schools of social work have a health concentration, and a few schools of public health have developed dual degree programs with schools of social work leading to a combined M.S.W./M.P.H. degree. The M.S.W. degree usually requires two years of work and the dual degree can be earned in three years.

The usual area of emphasis in schools of social work has centered on work in medical care settings. Recently, however, the community setting has attracted more emphasis and new curricula are emerging that include work in epidemiology and public health policy. Schools of social work have added a great deal of content in the health and public health areas in recent years. Social work content is not usually available in a school of public health curriculum, and students wishing to pursue a combined career will need to develop their social work content separately where dual degree programs or other collaborative arrangements do not exist.

OTHER CAREERS

There are many careers in public health and many different routes to those careers. This chapter has focused only on the careers most often available and needed. As has been noted earlier, virtually any legal profession or discipline has a public health role to play, from anthropology to zoology, from policy development and administration to water testing and hearing screening.

Many successful careers can be established with only the clinical skills required of the profession or discipline itself. But for those interested in a progressive career with the challenges and rewards that entails, education in public health is highly desirable.

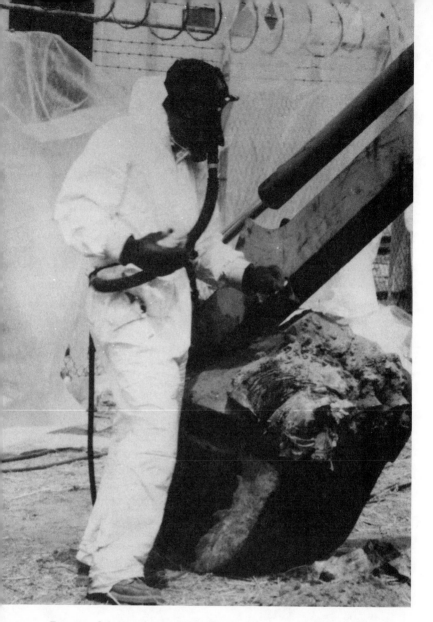

Because of the growing problem of hazardous materials in the workplace, industrial hygienists will play an important role in the future. (County of Los Angeles Department of Health Services photo)

CHAPTER 8

THE FUTURE OF PUBLIC HEALTH

The future of public health, as a concept, as a presence in every community, and as a career, is very much dependent on public attitudes in the United States. Does society expect its government to act on its behalf to prevent disease and disability, and, if so, to what extent?

If society's expectations were limited to those of the early nineteenth century, then the future of public health would be quite limited. Those expectations were of minimal government involvement in the affairs of a community or a business and reliance on the forces of the marketplace to produce both a robust and a healthy economy.

In the past decade we have witnessed a considerable reversion in attitudes in the United States toward that nineteenth century model. Yet while the public seemed to support reduced taxes and a decreased role for government, poll after poll indicated that people wanted environmental protection and available health services of high quality. Our society wants—demands—that our government take steps to protect us from hazards, even some of those we create for ourselves.

AN AMBIVALENT PUBLIC

Arthur Schlesinger, Sr., in 1949, predicted that the present conservative epoch would begin in 1978. Arthur Schlesinger, Jr., in

1986, suggested that the conservative cycle will begin to burn out in the 1980s with a return to more altruistic motivations in the 1990s and into the twenty-first century—just at the time when most people who are now contemplating college will be entering into the most productive years of their careers.

Too much can be made of cycles. In fact, public health careers suffered only a slight decline in the 1980s, as did many other public programs. But it is clear that many important things were lost during that time: immunization levels declined, the infant mortality rate rose, more people had less health insurance, and protection of workers from the hazards of their occupations decreased. The public seems unwilling to tolerate continued erosion of what have come to be considered derived rights in a civilized society. Public expectations are high as skepticism, but legislative bodies and governors throughout the country are more than willing, they are eager, to support well-thought-out, well-managed public health programs that will reduce the amount of disability and dependency in society.

The 1960s

A similar phenomenon occurred in the 1960s with the New Frontier of President Kennedy and the Great Society of President Johnson, but there was an important difference. At that time, the reality of scarce resources in this most affluent country was recognized by only a few people. We were convinced that we could conquer the moon, cancer, and poverty, and we set out to do all three with bold new programs, catapulting scant social experiments into national policy with large appropriations: the regional medical programs to conquer heart disease, cancer, and stroke; the Comprehensive Health Planning Program to assure all people access to high quality medical care; Medicare and Medicaid as the first steps toward a comprehensive national health insurance program; consolidated grants to provide comprehensive health services to mothers and children; nutrition programs to wipe out hunger. And, of course, we tried to fight a war at the same time.

Ten years later, the war was lost, people were still dying of cancer and heart disease and stroke, many people still could not obtain the medical care they needed, and the infant mortality rate had not declined. If anything, the problems have become worse since then.

The 1980s

The public is no longer willing to spend large amounts of money on programs it does not trust. But there are exceptions that point to the future of public health. In several states, governors have worked with coalitions of health leaders to develop new approaches to improving maternal and health care. In other states, thoughtful and creative new approaches to providing health care for the poor have been developed. In many states, with federal urging, seat belts have become mandatory. Areas in which people can smoke cigarettes have been restricted (and fewer people are smoking). Attitudes toward alcohol-related problems have become tougher and more realistic.

While the era has been confusing, certain messages are beginning to become apparent. Communities will tolerate, in fact they will insist upon, the careful implementation of well-thought-out programs with demonstrable benefits to their health. Moreover, they are willing to support well-managed programs to provide health services for the poor, not only through insurance schemes such as Medicare and Medicaid, but through the organization and utilization of public resources to actually produce and directly provide the needed services.

The message is neither liberal nor conservative, neither Democratic nor Republican: it is traditionally American, willing to experiment, willing to help, wanting to improve, a combination of beneficence and utilitarianism, insisting on prudent management by well-trained and knowledgeable professionals. As in all worthwhile careers, the future is very bright for those who are willing to take it seriously and learn how to manage it.

THE GOVERNMENTAL PRESENCE IN THE TWENTY-FIRST CENTURY

The Field Concept of Intervention

In 1974, the Canadian minister of health, the Honorable Marc LaLonde, published *The Health of Canadians,* in which he discussed the "field" concept of intervention. The causes of diseases and injuries can be found in one of four fields:

- The environmental field—includes traditional concerns, such as the supply of safe water and the effective disposal of sewage and garbage, as well as more modern problems such as asbestos in our buildings and dioxins in pesticides.
- The behavioral or life-style field—includes such obvious problems as tobacco use, drug abuse, and risk-taking behavior of adolescents.
- The biological field—includes our use of vaccines to induce immunity to serious diseases and the recent, explosive growth in the study of genetic predisposition to various diseases.
- The organizational field—includes the organization of emergency health services and the availability of prenatal care services for young women and other high-risk mothers-to-be.

Most of the common and important public health problems have their antecedent causes in more than one of the four fields.

For example, teenage pregnancy is primarily a problem attributed to the behavioral field. But it is clear that the problems of a high risk pregnancy in a young woman are also attributable to the environment in which she lives, the organization and availability of helping services, and her own biology. Smoking is a risk factor in pregnancy, as are dilapidated housing, atmospheric lead, diabetes, poor nutrition, and impeded access to acceptable health services. In which field should we concentrate our efforts?

High blood pressure is primarily a problem of the biological field, and not enough is known about why some people have it and others do not. Yet diet and exercise (the behavioral field) have an impact on high blood pressure, as does stress (the environment), and the availability and accessibility of good health services (the organization field).

If the risk factors and etiological antecedents for common and important diseases are carefully examined in each of the four fields, possible preventive interventions become evident. For example, a reduction of saturated fats in the diet, an increase in the proportion of complex carbohydrates, and a change from animal proteins to fish and poultry may have a significant effect on the prevalence of high blood pressure. Weight control and exercise also appear to exert a strong and beneficial effect. In addition, these preventive interventions have what are known as "cross-cutting" effects on other health problems such as diabetes, heart disease, and stroke. Such interventions suggest major new educational efforts, a change in agricultural research directions, and attempt to encourage different approaches to the use of leisure time. Public and private recreation programs are an important aspect of such efforts, as are changes in school lunch programs. Field intervention is a multi-faceted, multi-benefit approach to improved health and decreased dependency on medical care in treating single, established, persistently disabling diseases.

Medical Care vs. Public Health

Traditionally, the United States has attempted to concentrate on the organization and provision of direct medical care services to cope with health problems. We are proud of our medical care successes even if we complain about their cost and the apparent impersonality of the system. We have found it easier to approach the health problems of infancy and childhood with physicians and nurses and pills and shots than to organize public resources to intervene in the environmental and life-style fields.

One of the important differences between medical care and public health is the comprehensiveness of public health: rather than using only the tools of medicine, it will use whatever works and is acceptable to solve a problem. Public health engineers worked to fluoridate our water supplies rather than fill holes in teeth. Public health educators sought to reduce cigarette smoking rather than perfect surgical techniques to treat lung cancer. Environmental health workers have tried to remove asbestos from common usage rather than to treat a hopeless disease. Public health leaders worked to get seat belts and other protective devices more widely used rather than simply organize bigger and faster emergency medical care systems.

To the extent that the public, in its many communities, gradually recognizes that most of the serious health problems can be prevented by organized interventions, careers in public health will become increasingly challenging and fulfilling.

In each of the four fields (the environment, life-style, biology, and organizational), research and skillful management is resulting in stronger public support for appropriate interventions. At the present time, the federal government is wrestling with its major medical care programs: Medicaid and Medicare. Public health programs have received little attention.

Government Involvement

But the basic research structures are still in place and very active: the National Institutes of Health, the Centers for Disease Control, the Office of Health Research, Statistics and Technology, and the National Institute for Occupational Safety and Health. Many congressional leaders are eager to expand the federal government's role in prevention and health promotion. The primary restraints are the budget (a huge federal deficit coupled with large expenditures for medical care, social security, and defense) and a hesitancy to meddle too much in personal life-styles and other traditionally private matters at the national level—a hesitancy which is appropriate, given the propensity for large governments to make large mistakes.

At the state level, there often is a greater willingness to experiment. The states can more easily grasp a new notion and gain the support necessary for innovative attempts to prevent disease and injury. In recent years, the federal government has withdrawn from its acquired role as a major player in health policy formation, leaving the states to grapple with the complex and important problems of AIDS, maternal and child health, long-term care, medical care of the indigent, and environmental protection.

The states have many agencies with a role to play in public health: the state and local public health agencies principally, but also mental health agencies, substance abuse agencies, environmental protection agencies, occupational safety and health agencies, and departments of education, commerce, and agriculture. The need for trained health workers is increasing in the public sector at the state and local levels and will increase at the national level during the 1990s. Especially needed are people trained in epidemiology, toxicology, management, policy analysis, and disease prevention.

PROBLEM SOLVING IN THE FUTURE

The best training for a future career in public health is that which couples clinical training (such as nursing or medicine) with training in public health. Entry level jobs in public health that do not require college and postgraduate training will be less and less common. The health problems of the late twentieth century and the twenty-first century are too complex to allow simple solutions. They have their antecedents in more than one field, and their solutions will require skillful, multidisciplinary efforts. The public has shown that it is willing and eager to support such efforts when they are developed and managed by well-trained people who are dedicated to the public's interest.

In one sense, public health has a special capability for problem solving in the years ahead. As knowledge has expanded at an exponential rate, education and training programs have become increasingly specialized in order to provide people with a sense of personal control over their lives and to provide workers who can use the new technologies. Yet the important problems of the future are inherently complex and require the attention of many different disciplines working synergistically. This is difficult to accomplish, but public health has always been an interdisciplinary profession. As has been shown repeatedly in these chapters, the successes of public health were the result of leaders' ability to effectively harness the capabilities of many different people: to weave a warm tapestry out of the single threads of epidemiology, engineering, law, medicine, nursing, psychology, and management.

The power of future problem-solving efforts is dependent on the ability of people to pull together their careers rather than to separate them. That is what public health is all about.

PUBLIC HEALTH AND RELATED ORGANIZATIONS

The following organizations are good sources of information and statistics in their respective fields. Many also publish journals concerning information and issues of importance and interest to their organizations.

ACCREDITING COMMISSION ON EDUCATION FOR HEALTH
    SERVICES ADMINISTRATION
    Suite 503
    1911 North Fort Myer Drive
    Arlington, Virginia 22209

Evaluates and accredits graduate school programs in health services administration.

AMERICAN ASSOCIATION OF OCCUPATIONAL HEALTH NURSES
    Suite 400
    3500 Piedmont Road, N.E.
    Atlanta, Georgia 30305

Comprises professional nurses practicing in the field of occupational health nursing.

AMERICAN ASSOCIATION OF PUBLIC HEALTH DENTISTS
    223 Fontaine Circle
    Lexington, Kentucky 40506

Sponsors the development of opportunities for continuing education programs in dentistry.

AMERICAN ASSOCIATION OF PUBLIC HEALTH PHYSICIANS
P.O. Box 522
Greenwood, Mississippi 38930

Promotes physician leadership in public health.

AMERICAN COLLEGE OF PREVENTIVE MEDICINE
Suite 403
1015 15th Street, N.W.
Washington, D.C. 20005

Comprised of physicians who specialize in preventive medicine,
public health, occupational medicine, and aerospace medicine.

AMERICAN CONFERENCE OF GOVERNMENTAL INDUSTRIAL
HYGIENISTS, INC.
650 Glenway Avenue, Building D-5
Cincinnati, Ohio 45211

Includes industrial hygienists, physicians, nurses, and safety professionals employed by governmental agencies.

AMERICAN DENTAL ASSOCIATION
211 East Chicago Avenue
Chicago, Illinois 60611

Includes more than 140,000 dentists.

AMERICAN DIETETIC ASSOCIATION
430 North Michigan Avenue
Chicago, Illinois 60611

Comprises dieticians and nutritionists, 1,200 of whom are public
health nutritionists.

AMERICAN INDUSTRIAL HYGIENE ASSOCIATION
475 Wolf Ledges Parkway
Akron, Ohio 44311

Includes industrial hygienists employed in both the public and
private sectors.

AMERICAN MEDICAL ASSOCIATION
535 North Dearborn Street
Chicago, Illinois 60610

Collects and disseminates extensive data on all physicians in the
United States. Public health practitioners include aerospace med-

icine specialists, general preventive medicine specialists, occupational medicine specialists, and public health physicians.

AMERICAN NURSES ASSOCIATION
2420 Pershing Road
Kansas City, Missouri 64108

Comprised of approximately 164,600 members from all nursing areas including community health, gerontology, and occupational health.

AMERICAN PUBLIC HEALTH ASSOCIATION
1015 15th Street, N.W.
Washington, D.C. 20005

Includes all categories of public health personnel including public health physicians, nurses, nutritionists, social workers, epidemiologists, consultants, analysts, administrators, dentists, veterinarians, laboratory technicians, researchers, sanitarians, engineers, and planners.

AMERICAN VETERINARY MEDICAL ASSOCIATION
930 North Meacham Road
Schaumburg, Illinois 60172

Has more than 36,000 members representing between 80 and 85 percent of the veterinarians in the United States.

ASSOCIATION OF SCHOOLS OF PUBLIC HEALTH
Suite 404
1015 15th Street, N.W.
Washington, D.C. 20005

Comprised of accredited schools of public health.

ASSOCIATION OF STATE AND TERRITORIAL HEALTH OFFICIALS
Suite 207
10400 Connecticut Avenue
Kensington, Maryland 20895

Includes health directors from the states and territories of the United States. ASTHO has developed the National Public Health Program Reporting System (NPHPRS), which enables state health agencies to compare data.

ASSOCIATION OF UNIVERSITY PROGRAMS IN HEALTH
ADMINISTRATION
Suite 503
1911 North Fort Myer Drive
Arlington, Virginia 22209

Comprised of graduate and undergraduate programs in health administration. Conducts surveys of health administration programs including statistical, graduate placement, and faculty salary surveys.

CONFERENCE OF PUBLIC HEALTH LAB DIRECTORS
P.O. Box 9083
Austin, Texas 78766

Comprises individuals directing or assisting in directing public health laboratories, hospital labs, or research labs.

COUNCIL ON EDUCATION FOR PUBLIC HEALTH
1015 15th Street, N.W.
Washington, D.C. 20005

Evaluates and accredits schools of public health and graduate programs in health education and preventive or community medicine.

COUNCIL ON SOCIAL WORK EDUCATION
Suite 501
111 8th Avenue
New York, New York 10011

Concerned with the status and problems of social work education. Gathers data from graduating classes of schools of social work.

NATIONAL CENTER FOR HEALTH EDUCATION
211 Sutters Street, Fourth Floor
San Francisco, California 94108

Gathers and disseminates information pertaining to health education and health educators.

NATIONAL ENVIRONMENTAL HEALTH ASSOCIATION
Suite 704
1200 Lincoln Street
Denver, Colorado 80203

Comprises those working in environmental health for governmental health agencies, public health education, or inspection services for private employers. The NEHA has an undergraduate scholarship program.

NATIONAL LEAGUE FOR NURSING
  10 Columbus Circle
  New York, New York 10019

Gathers and disseminates data pertaining to the nursing profession. Accredits schools and programs of nursing.

SOCIETY FOR EPIDEMIOLOGIC RESEARCH
  c/o American Journal of Epidemiology
  550 North Broadway
  Baltimore, Maryland 21205

Comprises epidemiologists, researchers, public health administrators, statisticians, mathematicians, and others interested in epidemiological research.

FEDERAL PUBLIC HEALTH AGENCIES

CENTERS FOR DISEASE CONTROL
  Department of Health and Human Services
  Building 1, Room B63
  1600 Clifton Road, N.E.
  Atlanta, Georgia 30333

NATIONAL INSTITUTE OF OCCUPATIONAL SAFETY AND
  HEALTH
  255 East Paces Ferry Road, N.E.
  Atlanta, Georgia 30305

NATIONAL INSTITUTES OF HEALTH
  Building 31, Room 2B-10
  9000 Rockville Pike
  Bethesda, Maryland 20892

UNITED STATES PUBLIC HEALTH SERVICE
  Department of Health and Human Services
  Room 716G
  200 Independence Avenue, S.W.
  Washington, D.C. 20201

STATE PUBLIC HEALTH AGENCIES

Every state has a state public health association, and almost all of them are affiliated with the American Public Health Association, the oldest and largest public health association in the world. The mailing address changes from year to year depending on who the elected officers are. They can usually be contacted by asking people in the local or state health department how to get in touch with them.

In addition to the following agencies, there are local health departments in almost every community of the United States. They can be found under the city or county office listings. In those states without local health departments, look in the state listings.

ALABAMA DEPARTMENT OF PUBLIC HEALTH
   381 State Office Building
   Montgomery, Alabama 36130

ALASKA DEPARTMENT OF HEALTH AND SOCIAL SERVICES
   Division of Public Health
   P.O. Box H-06
   Juneau, Alaska 99811

AMERICAN SAMOA DEPARTMENT OF HEALTH
   Government of American Samoa
   Pago Pago, American Samoa 96799

ARIZONA DEPARTMENT OF HEALTH SERVICES
   1740 West Adams Street
   Phoenix, Arizona 85007

ARKANSAS DEPARTMENT OF HEALTH
4815 West Markham Street
Little Rock, Arkansas 72201

CALIFORNIA STATE DEPARTMENT OF HEALTH SERVICES
714 P Street, Room 1253
Sacramento, California 95814

COLORADO DEPARTMENT OF HEALTH
4210 East 11th Avenue
Denver, Colorado 80220

CONNECTICUT DEPARTMENT OF HEALTH SERVICES
150 Washington Street
Hartford, Connecticut 06106

DELAWARE DEPARTMENT OF HEALTH AND SOCIAL SERVICES
Division of Public Health
Robbins Building
802 Silver Lake Boulevard and Walker Road
Dover, Delaware 19901

DISTRICT OF COLUMBIA DEPARTMENT OF HUMAN SERVICES
Division of Public Health
1875 Connecticut Avenue, N.W., Room 825
Washington, D.C. 20009

FLORIDA DEPARTMENT OF HEALTH AND REHABILITATIVE
SERVICES
1323 Winewood Boulevard
Tallahassee, Florida 32301

GEORGIA DEPARTMENT OF HUMAN RESOURCES
Division of Public Health
878 Peachtree Street, Room 201, N.E.
Atlanta, Georgia 30309

GUAM DEPARTMENT OF PUBLIC HEALTH AND SOCIAL
SERVICES
P.O. Box 2816
Agana, Guam 96910

HAWAII DEPARTMENT OF HEALTH
Kinau Hale, P.O. Box 3378
Honolulu, Hawaii 96801

IDAHO DEPARTMENT OF HEALTH AND WELFARE
  Division of Health
  Statehouse Mall
  Boise, Idaho 83720

ILLINOIS DEPARTMENT OF PUBLIC HEALTH
  535 West Jefferson Street
  Springfield, Illinois 62761

INDIANA STATE BOARD OF HEALTH
  1330 West Michigan Street
  P.O. Box 1964
  Indianapolis, Indiana 46206

IOWA DEPARTMENT OF HEALTH
  Lucas State Office Building
  Des Moines, Iowa 50319

KANSAS DEPARTMENT OF HEALTH AND ENVIRONMENT
  Division of Health
  Forbes Field
  Topeka, Kansas 66620

KENTUCKY CABINET FOR HUMAN RESOURCES
  Bureau for Health Services
  275 East Main Street
  Frankfort, Kentucky 40621

LOUISIANA DEPARTMENT OF HEALTH AND HUMAN
  RESOURCES
  Office of Preventive and Public Health Services
  P.O. Box 60630
  New Orleans, Louisiana 70160

MAINE DEPARTMENT OF HUMAN SERVICES
  Bureau of Health
  Augusta, Maine 04333

MARYLAND DEPARTMENT OF HEALTH AND MENTAL HYGIENE
  201 West Preston Street
  Baltimore, Maryland 21201

MASSACHUSETTS EXECUTIVE OFFICE OF HUMAN SERVICES
  Division of Public Health
  150 Tremont Street
  Boston, Massachusetts 02111

MICHIGAN DEPARTMENT OF PUBLIC HEALTH
3500 North Logan Street
Lansing, Michigan 48909

MINNESOTA DEPARTMENT OF HEALTH
717 Delaware Street, S.E.
Minneapolis, Minnesota 55440

MISSISSIPPI STATE BOARD OF HEALTH
P.O. Box 1700
Jackson, Mississippi 39205

MISSOURI DEPARTMENT OF HEALTH
P.O. Box 570
Jefferson City, Missouri 65102

MONTANA DEPARTMENT OF HEALTH AND
ENVIRONMENTAL SCIENCES
Cogswell Building
Helena, Montana 59620

NEBRASKA DEPARTMENT OF HEALTH
301 Centennial Mall South
Lincoln, Nebraska 68509

NEVADA DEPARTMENT OF HUMAN RESOURCES
505 East King Street
Capitol Complex
Carson City, Nevada 89710

NEW HAMPSHIRE DIVISION OF PUBLIC HEALTH
SERVICES/DEPARTMENT OF HEALTH AND HUMAN SERVICES
Health and Welfare Building
6 Hazen Drive
Concord, New Hampshire 03301-6527

NEW JERSEY DEPARTMENT OF HEALTH
CN 360, John Fitch Plaza
Trenton, New Jersey 08625

NEW MEXICO HEALTH AND ENVIRONMENT DEPARTMENT
P.O. Box 968
Santa Fe, New Mexico 87504-0968

NEW YORK DEPARTMENT OF HEALTH
Empire State Plaza
Corning Tower Building
Albany, New York 12237

NORTH CAROLINA DEPARTMENT OF HUMAN RESOURCES
    Division of Health Services
    P.O. Box 2091
    Raleigh, North Carolina 27602

NORTH DAKOTA STATE DEPARTMENT OF HEALTH
    State Capitol
    Bismarck, North Dakota 58505

NORTHERN MARIANA ISLANDS DEPARTMENT OF PUBLIC
    HEALTH AND ENVIRONMENTAL SERVICES
    Saipan, CM 96950

OHIO DEPARTMENT OF HEALTH
    246 North High Street
    P.O. Box 118
    Columbus, Ohio 43266-0588

OKLAHOMA STATE DEPARTMENT OF HEALTH
    P.O. Box 53551
    Oklahoma City, Oklahoma 73152

OREGON DEPARTMENT OF HUMAN RESOURCES
    State Health Division
    811 State Office Building, P.O. Box 231
    Portland, Oregon 97207

PENNSYLVANIA DEPARTMENT OF HEALTH
    P.O. Box 90
    Harrisburg, Pennsylvania 17120

PUERTO RICO DEPARTMENT OF HEALTH
    Building A
    San Juan, Puerto Rico 00936

RHODE ISLAND DEPARTMENT OF HEALTH
    Cannon Building, 75 Davis Street
    Providence, Rhode Island 02908

SOUTH CAROLINA DEPARTMENT OF HEALTH AND
    ENVIRONMENTAL CONTROL
    2600 Bull Street
    Columbia, South Carolina 29201

SOUTH DAKOTA DEPARTMENT OF HEALTH
    Joe Foss Building, 523 East Capitol
    Pierre, South Dakota 57501

TENNESSEE DEPARTMENT OF HEALTH AND ENVIRONMENT
344 Cordell Hull Building
Nashville, Tennessee 37219

TEXAS DEPARTMENT OF HEALTH
1100 West 49th Street
Austin, Texas 78756

TRUST TERRITORY OF THE PACIFIC ISLANDS
OFFICE OF HEALTH SERVICES
Saipan, Mariana Islands 96950

UTAH DEPARTMENT OF HEALTH
P.O. Box 45500
Salt Lake City, Utah 84145-0500

VERMONT DEPARTMENT OF HEALTH
60 Main Street
P.O. Box 70
Burlington, Vermont 05402

VIRGINIA STATE HEALTH DEPARTMENT
109 Governor Street
Richmond, Virginia 23219

VIRGIN ISLAND DEPARTMENT OF HEALTH
P.O. Box 7309
St. Thomas, Virgin Islands 00801

WASHINGTON DEPARTMENT OF SOCIAL AND HEALTH
SERVICES
Division of Health
Mail Stop ET-21
Olympia, Washington 98504

WEST VIRGINIA DEPARTMENT OF HEALTH
Building 3, Room 206
State Capitol Complex
Charleston, West Virginia 25305

WISCONSIN DIVISION OF HEALTH
1 West Wilson Street
P.O. Box 309
Madison, Wisconsin 53701

WYOMING HEALTH AND MEDICAL SERVICES
Hathaway Building
Cheyenne, Wyoming 82002

UNITED STATES SCHOOLS OF PUBLIC HEALTH AND GRADUATE PUBLIC HEALTH PROGRAMS

The following schools of public health and graduate public health programs were accredited in 1987 by the Council on Education for Public Health.

Schools of Public Health

University of Alabama at Birmingham School of Public Health
    University Station
    Birmingham, Alabama 35294

Boston University School of Public Health
    School of Medicine
    80 East Concord Street
    Boston, Massachusetts 02118

University of California at Berkeley School of Public Health
    19 Earl Warren Hall
    Berkeley, California 94720

University of California at Los Angeles School of Public Health
    Center for the Health Sciences
    Los Angeles, California 90024

Columbia University School of Public Health
    600 West 168th Street
    New York, New York 10032

Harvard University School of Public Health
    677 Huntington Avenue
    Boston, Massachusetts 02115

University of Hawaii School of Public Health
    1960 East-West Road
    Honolulu, Hawaii 96822

University of Illinois at Chicago School of Public Health
    Health Sciences Center
    P.O. Box 6998
    Chicago, Illinois 60680

The Johns Hopkins University School of Hygiene and Public Health
    615 North Wolfe Street
    Baltimore, Maryland 21205

Loma Linda University School of Health
    Loma Linda, California 92350

University of Massachusetts Division of Public Health
    School of Health Sciences
    Amherst, Massachusetts 01003-0037

University of Michigan School of Public Health
    109 South Observatory Street
    Ann Arbor, Michigan 48109

University of Minnesota School of Public Health
    1360 Mayo Memorial Building
    420 Delaware Street, S.E.
    Minneapolis, Minnesota 55455-0318

University of North Carolina School of Public Health
    Rosenau Hall 201-H
    Chapel Hill, North Carolina 27514

University of Oklahoma College of Public Health
    Health Sciences Center
    P.O. Box 26901
    Oklahoma City, Oklahoma 73190

University of Pittsburgh Graduate School of Public Health
    111 Parran Hall
    Pittsburgh, Pennsylvania 15261

University of Puerto Rico School of Public Health
  Medical Sciences Campus
  G.P.O. Box 5067
  San Juan, Puerto Rico 00936

San Diego State University Graduate School of Public Health
  College of Human Services
  San Diego, California 92182

University of South Carolina School of Public Health
  College of Health
  Columbia, South Carolina 29208

University of Texas School of Public Health
  Health Science Center at Houston
  P.O. Box 20186
  Houston, Texas 77025

Tulane University School of Public Health and Tropical Medicine
  1430 Tulane Avenue
  New Orleans, Louisiana 70112

University of Washington School of Public Health and Community
  Medicine
  F356d Health Sciences Building
  Mail Drop SC-30
  Seattle, Washington 98195

Yale University Department of Epidemiology and Public Health
  School of Medicine
  P.O. Box 3333
  60 College Street
  New Haven, Connecticut 06510

Graduate Programs in Community Health Education

California State University–Northridge MPH Program in Community
  Health Education, Department of Health Science
  School of Communication and Professional Studies
  18111 Nordhoff Street
  Northridge, California 91330

Hunter College Community Health Education Program
  School of Health Sciences
  425 East 25th Street
  New York, New York 10010

University of Illinois at Urbana–Champaign Community Health
Education Program
Department of Health and Safety Studies
1206 South 4th Street
Champaign, Illinois 61820

New York University MPH Program in Community Health Education
Department of Health Education, School of Education, Health, Nursing
and Arts Professions
715 Broadway
Second Floor
Washington Square
New York, New York 10003

San Jose State University MPH Program in Community Health Education
Department of Health Science
School of Applied Sciences and Arts
San Jose, California 95192

Temple University Master of Public Health Program
College of Health, Physical Education, Recreation and Dance
Philadelphia, Pennsylvania 19122

University of Tennessee MPH Program in Community Health Education
Division of Public Health
School of Health, Physical Education and Recreation
Knoxville, Tennessee 37996-2700

Graduate Programs in Community Health/Preventive Medicine

University of Colorado Masters Program in Preventive Medicine
Department of Preventive Medicine and Biometrics
Health Sciences Center
Campus Box C-245
4200 East 9th Avenue
Denver, Colorado 80262

University of Connecticut Master of Science in Community Health
Program
Department of Community Medicine and Health Care
School of Medicine
Farmington, Connecticut 06032

Emory University Master of Public Health Program
  School of Medicine
  Department of Community Health
  735 Gatewood Road, N.E.
  Atlanta, Georgia 30322

University of Miami Master of Public Health and Master of Science
  Public Health Programs
  Department of Epidemiology and Public Health
  School of Medicine
  P.O. Box 016069
  Miami, Florida 33101

University of Medicine and Dentistry of New Jersey–Rutgers, The State
  University of New Jersey Graduate Program in Public Health
  Department of Environmental and Community Medicine
  Piscataway, New Jersey 08854

Ohio State University Graduate Program in Preventive Medicine and
  Community Health
  Department of Preventive Medicine
  School of Medicine
  Starling Loving Hall
  Columbus, Ohio 43210-1228

University of Rochester Master of Science in Community Health Program
  School of Medicine and Dentistry
  601 Elmwood Avenue
  Rochester, New York 14642

St. Louis University Graduate Program in Community Health
  Center for Health Services Education and Research
  Medical Center
  3525 Caroline Street
  St. Louis, Missouri 63104

Uniformed Services University of the Health Sciences MPH and MTM&H
  Graduate Programs
  4301 Jones Bridge Road
  Bethesda, Maryland 20814

University of Utah Master of Science in Public Health
  Department of Family and Preventive Medicine
  Medical Center
  50 North Medical Drive
  Salt Lake City, Utah 84132

APPENDIX E

REFERENCES

American Public Health Association. "The Role of Official Local Health Agencies." *American Journal of Public Health* 65 (1975): 189.

American Public Health Association, the Association of State and Territorial Health Officials, the National Association of County Health Officials, the United States Conference of Local Health Officers, and the Centers for Disease Control of the United States Public Health Service. *Model Standards: A Guide for Community Preventive Health Services.* 2d ed. Washington, D.C.: American Public Health Association, 1985.

Behneman, H.M.F. "Leaves from a Doctor's Notebook of Seventy Years Ago." *Military Surgeon* 86 (June 1940): 547.

Butter, I., E. Carpenter, B. Kay, and R. Simmons. *Sex and Status: Hierarchies in the Health Workforce.* School of Public Health, Department of Health Planning and Administration, Public Health Policy Series. Ann Arbor: The University of Michigan Press, 1985.

Garrison, F.H. *An Introduction to the History of Medicine.* 4th ed. Philadelphia: W.B. Saunders Company, 1929.

George, M.D. *London Life in the Eighteenth Century.* New York: Alfred A. Knopf, 1925.

Hanlon, J.J. and G.E. Pickett. *Public Health: Administration and Practice.* 8th ed. St. Louis: Times/Mirror Mosby, 1984.

Holmes, O.W. *Medical Essays.* In *Writings,* vol. 9. Boston: Houghton Mifflin Company, 1891.

Jensen, H.E. "Mental Health: A Local Public Health Responsibility." *Mental Hygiene* 37 (October 1953): 530.

LaLonde, M. *A New Perspective on the Health of Canadians: A Working Document.* Ottawa: Ministry of National Health and Welfare, 1974.

Public Health Agencies, 1987: Expenditures and Sources of Funds. Washington, D.C.: The Public Health Foundation.

Ravenal, M.P., ed. *A Half Century of Public Health.* New York: American Public Health Association, 1921.

Richardson, B.W. *The Health of Nations: A Review of the Works of Edwin Chadwick.* vol. 2. London: Longmans Green and Company, 1887.

Shattuck, Lemuel. *Report of the Sanitary Commission of Massachusetts.* 1850. Reprint. Cambridge: Harvard University Press, 1948.

Starr, Paul. *The Social Transformation of American Medicine.* New York: Basic Books, Inc., 1982.

U.S. Department of Health and Human Services. *The Fifth Report to the President and the Congress on the Status of Health Personnel in the United States.* Washington, D.C., March 1986.

———. 1984. *Minorities and Women in the Health Fields.* Publication no. (HRSA) HRS-DV 84-5. Washington, D.C., September.

Winslow, C.E.A. "The Untilled Field of Public Health." *Modern Medicine* 2 (March 1920): 183.

VGM CAREER BOOKS

OPPORTUNITIES IN

Available in both paperback and hardbound editions

Accounting Careers
Acting Careers
Advertising Careers
Agriculture Careers
Airline Careers
Animal and Pet Care
Appraising Valuation Science
Architecture
Automotive Service
Banking
Beauty Culture
Biological Sciences
Book Publishing Careers
Broadcasting Careers
Building Construction Trades
Business Communication Careers
Business Management
Cable Television
Carpentry Careers
Chemical Engineering
Chemistry Careers
Child Care Careers
Chiropractic Health Care
Civil Engineering Careers
Commercial Art and Graphic Design
Computer Aided Design and Computer Aided Mfg.
Computer Maintenance Careers
Computer Science Careers
Counseling & Development
Crafts Careers
Dance
Data Processing Careers
Dental Care
Drafting Careers
Electrical Trades
Electronic and Electrical Engineering
Energy Careers
Engineering Technology Careers
Environmental Careers
Fashion Careers
Federal Government Careers
Film Careers
Financial Careers
Fire Protection Services
Fitness Careers
Food Services
Foreign Language Careers
Forestry Careers
Gerontology Careers
Government Service
Graphic Communications
Health and Medical Careers

High Tech Careers
Home Economics Careers
Hospital Administration
Hotel & Motel Management
Industrial Design
Insurance Careers
Interior Design
Journalism Careers
Landscape Architecture
Law Careers
Law Enforcement and Criminal Justice
Library and Information Science
Machine Trades
Magazine Publishing Careers
Management
Marine & Maritime Careers
Marketing Careers
Materials Science
Mechanical Engineering
Microelectronics
Modeling Careers
Music Careers
Nursing Careers
Nutrition Careers
Occupational Therapy Careers
Office Occupations
Opticianry
Optometry
Packaging Science
Paralegal Careers
Paramedical Careers
Part-time & Summer Jobs
Personnel Management
Pharmacy Careers
Photography
Physical Therapy Careers
Podiatric Medicine
Printing Careers
Psychiatry
Psychology
Public Health Careers
Public Relations Careers
Real Estate
Recreation and Leisure
Refrigeration and Air Conditioning
Religious Service
Robotics Careers
Sales Careers
Sales & Marketing
Secretarial Careers
Securities Industry
Social Work Careers
Speech-Language Pathology Careers
Sports & Athletics
Sports Medicine
State and Local Government

Teaching Careers
Technical Communications
Telecommunications
Television and Video Careers
Theatrical Design & Production
Transportation Careers
Travel Careers
Veterinary Medicine Careers
Vocational and Technical Careers
Word Processing
Writing Careers
Your Own Service Business

WOMEN IN

Communications
Engineering
Finance
Government
Management
Science
Their Own Business

CAREERS IN

Accounting
Business
Communications
Computers
Health Care
Science

CAREER DIRECTORIES

Careers Encyclopedia
Occupational Outlook Handbook

CAREER PLANNING

How to Get and Get Ahead On Your First Job
How to Get People to Do Things Your Way
How to Have a Winning Job Interview
How to Land a Better Job
How to Write a Winning Résumé
Joyce Lain Kennedy's Career Book
Life Plan
Planning Your Career Change
Planning Your Career of Tomorrow
Planning Your College Education
Planning Your Military Career
Planning Your Own Home Business
Planning Your Young Child's Education

SURVIVAL GUIDES

High School Survival Guide
College Survival Guide

 VGM Career Horizons
A Division of National Textbook Company
4255 West Touhy Avenue
Lincolnwood, Illinois 60646-1975 U.S.A.